To: Professor e

Dear Azeem,

For your expert comments!

Albert Lee

15 Feb 2010

Diagnosis and Management in Primary Care

A Problem-based Approach

EDITED BY

William C. W. Wong
Martin Lindsay
Albert Lee

The Chinese University Press

Diagnosis and Management in Primary Care:
A Problem-based Approach
William C. W. Wong, Martin Lindsay and Albert Lee

© **The Chinese University of Hong Kong**, 2008

ISBN: 978–962–996–333–0

THE CHINESE UNIVERSITY PRESS
The Chinese University of Hong Kong
SHA TIN, N.T., HONG KONG
Fax: +852 2603 6692
    +852 2603 7355
E-mail: cup@cuhk.edu.hk
Web-site: www.chineseupress.com

Printed in Hong Kong

Contents

I. Principles of Diagnosis and Management

II. Problem-based Diagnoses and Management in the General Population

III. Problem-based Diagnoses and Management in the Specific Groups

IV. Self-assessment

Foreword

Family medicine is a key component of the healthcare system: from a medical generalistic perspective it assesses health problems, people in the community being consulted for, and prescribes treatment. This generalistic approach guarantees that medical care becomes effective, (cost) effective, timely and safe for patients.

The unique contribution of family medicine can be captured in terms of a holistic, personal approach to the health of people and their families. Continuity of care over time and integrating the knowledge of medical, psychological and social aspects of health shape this approach.

More than 90% of all professionally treated health problems are dealt with in family practice, and it is obvious that family practice is all about applying knowledge and skills. But family medicine is much more than the mere application of knowledge and skills of special domains of medical science, and here lies the great value of this book: it brings together the intellectual wisdom that shapes medical care in its personal orientation, taking into account the physical, environmental and psychological factors that determine illness and disease. The authors and editors deserve our greatest respect for the way in which they have brought the book together.

The book is a testimony of the international scientific basis of family medicine, and it will help students of medicine to find their way through the most difficult, the most demanding, but also the most exciting aspect of medical care, that of the family doctor.

The knowledge presented is of course important for students who are themselves pursuing a career in family practice. But even more important this knowledge is, it seems, for those who will practise in other clinical specialties, because the future of medical care makes it imperative to exploit the contribution of family practice to its full stretch, in order to cope with the challenges of modern health care: a measured response to the needs of an ageing population, and particular of the frail elderly with multiple chronic health problems depends on medical practitioners to demonstrate clinical competence and the ability to relate to the person of the patient over long periods of time. This requires the involvement of primary care, also for treatment initiated in the hospital.

I have little doubt that students, irrespective of their current or future career choice will find this book an indispensable companion for their studies.

Chris van Weel
Professor of Family Medicine and Head of
Department of Primary Care
Radboud University Medical Centre, Nijmegen, The Netherlands
President of the World Organization of Family Doctors (Wonca)

Foreword

⸎

Family medicine is well recognised as one of the most important disciplines in the medical field. According to the World Organization of Family Doctors, a family doctor is defined as a specialist trained to provide health care services for all individuals regardless of age, sex or type of health problem; to provide primary and continuous care for every family within the community; to address all kinds of physical, psychological and social problems; and to coordinate with other specialists to deliver comprehensive health care services when needed.

In other words, a family doctor takes care of all types of patients and handles all kinds of health problems in the community. One could understand the breadth of knowledge required for family doctors to carry out their duties. In the undergraduate curriculum, it is pivotal for students to understand the role of family doctors in the health care system as well as the interactions between the physical, social and psychological factors in the context of patient, family and the community.

This book covers general principles of family medicine in clinical practice. Consultation skills, psychological influences, diagnosis formulation, patient counselling, medico-legal problems and working relationships with non-governmental organisations are important issues in a primary care setting. This book allows its readers to gain thorough understanding of these topics, which is essential for developing a clinical sense in order to provide comprehensive and continuing patient care. Being acquainted with family medicine will prepare an individual to become a clinician, who chooses family medicine as a future career or partners with family doctors in patient management.

In addition, this book includes practical problem-based topics which family doctors commonly encounter in their actual practices. Although similar topics might be covered in other standard textbooks, this book presents the views of family doctors, and particularly from the angle of out-patient care. It is also a unique feature of this book that most chapters are written by local scholars who are most appropriate in giving the readers an overview of their experiences in local scenarios.

Disease patterns, acceptance of treatment and perception of sickness are heavily influenced by local culture, social ecology as well as the government health care policy. This book provides answers for questions unique to the local society that international textbooks could hardly address. This is an unprecedented family medicine textbook written by local scholars in Hong Kong. This book delineates clinical pictures specifically relevant to local family doctors. I am sure it will serve as a useful text for undergraduates and a valuable guide for trainees in family medicine.

Ip Kit-kuen, Andrew
MBBS (HK) MScSEM (Bath) FHKCFP FRACGP
FHKAM (Family Medicine) DCH (London) DOM (CUHK)
President, Hong Kong College of Family Physicians

Preface

Family medicine, once again, comes under the spotlight in the health care reform in Hong Kong following the publication of the Discussion Paper "Building a Healthy Tomorrow" in 2005. This paper highlighted the important roles of family doctors in our future healthcare system. In fact, roughly half of our local graduates practise family medicine, either in the private or the public sector, and invariably the other half utilise many family medicine skills such as consultation skills or diagnostic techniques and require communicating with their family medicine colleagues in their day-to-day work.

Nevertheless the undergraduate curriculum remains mainly system-based and hospital-orientated. From our teaching experience we find that many junior students have great difficulties when presented with a symptom or sign instead of a conventional disease category and nomenclature. How to extract the appropriate essential information, use what have been learnt in pre-clinical years, and then think laterally to make a clinical decision, remains a puzzle to many students when diving into the immense field of family medicine! Let alone the formulation of a management plan after a mere 10 minutes of consultation whilst taking into consideration the various psychosocial, medico-legal and cultural factors. Remember—the commitment of a family doctor is to "a person", not to "a disease" or to "a person with a certain disease".

The idea behind this new book is to provide clinical students with some basic principles of diagnosis and management, information on medico-legal pitfalls and the role of evidence in primary care. Then, using practical examples, we will take them through the mental process involved in coming to a clinical diagnosis, highlighting the important signs or symptoms and advising which investigations to request and why. In the management section we will use initial examples and guide them through the complexity of the disease as it progresses. Emphasis will be placed on how primary and secondary care coordinates. For example, the appearance of some "red flag" signs or symptoms when an urgent referral is required, and how and why a family doctor would select a particular drug for an individual patient, instead of giving a blanket cover of all the different classes of drugs for that condition as is given in most medical textbooks. Evidence-based medicine is an inevitable part of our management plans and some non-pharmacological treatment will also be discussed.

There are two clinical sections in this book: one on common diseases and the other on important diseases in specific "life cycle" groups such as men, women or children. The book deals with conditions that are common in this population and context. However the range of conditions covered is by no means exhaustive and this book should be used in conjunction with a sound medical textbook. It only serves to introduce students on how to apply knowledge in practical life situations and problem-based learning in the family medicine setting, where resources and facilities are often limited. There are exercises with some suggested answers in the last section so that students can practise their newly acquired skills.

I would like to take this opportunity to thank my co-editors and all the contributors for their tremendous support and commitment, and to acknowledge their contributions of wisdom, expertise, experience and passion. Without them, the compilation of this book would have been simply impossible. Together, we hope we can share our joy in family medicine and make it more exciting to the students.

William C. W. Wong
MB ChB MA MPH MD DFFP DCH DHCL
FRCAGP FRCGP MTFM RCSP
Associate Professor
February 2007

The Editors

꧁

❖ Associate Professor William Chi Wai **Wong**, MB, ChB, MA (Dist), MPH, MD, DFFP, DCH, DHCL, FRCGP, FRCAGP, MFTM, RCSP

Professor Wong was Associate Professor in the Department of Community and Family Medicine at The Chinese University of Hong Kong. He became the Director of General Practice and Primary Care Education at the University of Melbourne in December 2007. He graduated from the University of Edinburgh in 1993 and has extensive clinical experience working in Scotland, England, Australia, Hong Kong and China. His main research interests are sexual health, gender and health, and alternative medicine. He works closely with the social science disciplines applying both qualitative and quantitative research methodology in medicine. He has published over 60 papers including randomised controlled trials, prescribing patterns and clinical behaviours during SARS since he joined The Chinese University of Hong Kong in 2002. The results of these researches were disseminated to the general public through 32 newspaper reports and 2 radio (including *BBC World Service*) and 3 TV interviews.

❖ Dr. Martin Stephen **Lindsay**, MB, BS

Dr. Lindsay has practised primary care medicine in excess of 20 years. He has been instrumental in developing a leading multi-specialty primary care practice in an ethnically diverse and low socioeconomic inner city area of London. He has special interests in respiratory medicine and mental health.

He is a hospital practitioner in the Respiratory Department at The North Middlesex University (Teaching) Hospital. This also includes giving lectures to junior doctors. He collaborates with hospital colleagues to provide guidelines and to improve local services in respiratory medicine. He also provides advice to the London Strategic Health Authority and is on the advisory panel to the *Drug and Therapeutics Bulletin*.

Dr. Lindsay is a tutor to undergraduate medical students from University College and Royal Free Hospital Medical Schools in mental health. He is an MB, BS, final year medical examiner at University College and Royal Free Hospital Medical Schools and a trainer for Foundation Year 2 doctors. He is also the mental health lead for his Practice Based Commissioning Group and provides regular sessional work for the Drug Advisory Service in Haringey.

From February to July 2003 Dr. Lindsay spent a sabbatical at the Department of Community and Family Medicine in The Chinese University of Hong Kong.

❖ Professor Albert **Lee**, MB, BS (Lond), MPH, MD (CUHK), FRCP (Irel), FRACGP (Aus), FFPH (UK), FHKAM (Family Medicine), FHK, CFP, DCH

Professor Lee is Professor and Head of Division of Family Medicine and Primary Care of the Department of Community and Family Medicine and Director of the Centre for Health Education and Health Promotion of The Chinese University of Hong Kong. He is also the Honorary Consultant in Family Medicine and Head of Lek Yuen Family Medicine Health Centre. He has been appointed as Director of the Centre for General Practice Research Development of the Institute of Hospital Management of the Ministry of Health, China and Adjunct Professor of the Centre for Environmental and Population Health of Griffiths University, Australia since 2007. He was elected as one of the Global Vice President (2010 World Conference) of International Union for Health Promotion and Education (2007–2010).

Professor Lee received his medical degree at the University of London with various awards and merit certificates in 1984. He pursued further postgraduate studies with Diploma in Child Health at Royal College of Physicians and Surgeons in Ireland, Master of Public Health and Doctorate degree in Medicine (higher medical research degree MD: dissertation on health services research in primary care) at The Chinese University of Hong Kong, and also Diploma in Epidemiology and Biostatistics. He has been awarded Fellows of Royal College of Physicians of Ireland, Royal Australian College of General Practitioners, Faculty of Public Health of Royal College of Physicians of United Kingdom, Hong Kong Academy of Medicine (Family Medicine) and Hong Kong College of Family Physician. His clinical specialty is family medicine and his research area of interest is family and community health with special interests in child and adolescent health, primary care health services research, primary care management of chronic disease, comprehensive school health programme, medical education, and health education and health promotion. He has published over 140 papers in peer-reviewed journals and has been invited as a speaker in many international conferences. His work in community health is well recognised by the World Health Organization (WHO) and he has been invited by WHO to become temporary advisor on several occasions and has been commissioned by WHO Regional Office to conduct international workshops for other Asian and Pacific countries on school health. He started the first Master Degree and Postgraduate Diploma in Family Medicine and Health Education and Health Promotion in Hong Kong. He received the award for Chief Executive Commendation for Community Services in 2004 Honours list of Hong Kong SAR Government.

List of Contributors

❖ Dr. Andy Kit Ying **Cheung**, MBBS, DCH, DFM, FHK, CFP, FRACGP, FHKAM (Family Medicine), MSocSc (Couns)

Dr. Cheung is a family physician in private practice. She is also an adjunct Associate Professor in Family Medicine at The Chinese University of Hong Kong, Honorary Assistant Professor in Family Medicine at The University of Hong Kong and Honorary Lecturer at the Family Institute of the University of Hong Kong. Her main interest is in psychological medicine and integration of psychotherapeutic strategies in clinical practice. She has published articles on doctor-patient relationship, benefits of support groups for patients with depression, partner abuse and other topics.

❖ Dr. Gabriel Kin **Choi**, MB, LMCC, MRCS, MFM, MRCP, FRCPI, FRACGP, FACTM, FHKAM (Medicine), FHKAM (Family Medicine), DPD, DFM, DCH, DOM, DGM, PDID, PDCPM, PDCG

Dr. Choi is the current President of the Hong Kong Medical Association and Regional Advisor for the Royal College of Physicians of Ireland. He is a member of the Medical Council and has sat in 70 disciplinary inquiries and chaired two of them.

Dr. Choi graduated from The University of Hong Kong in 1972 with distinction in Preventive and Social Medicine. He was awarded Sir Robert Black Scholarship and trained in nephrology under Professor de Wardener of Charing Cross Hospital and A. J. Rees of Hammersmith Hospital in London. He was introduced to the discipline of family medicine at the University of Toronto when he arrived in Canada in 1989. He is currently Honorary Clinical Associate Professor of The Chinese University of Hong Kong and examiner for the RACGP/HKCFP conjoint examination. Prior to taking up the presidency of the Medical Association, he was a part-time consultant in family medicine in the Hospital Authority.

❖ Dr. Antonio An Tung **Chuh**, MBBS (HK), MD (HK), MRCP (UK), FRCP (Edin), FRCP ((Irel), FRCGP, FRACGP, FHKCFP, MFM (Monash), FHKAM (Family Medicine), DFM (Monash), DCH (Lond), DCH (Irel), DCCH (Edin), DipDerm (Glasg), Dip G-U Med (LAS)

Dr. Chuh is a part-time Associate Professor in the Department of Community and Family Medicine at The Chinese University of Hong Kong. He graduated from The University of Hong Kong in 1991 with the Dr. Sun Yat Sen Prize in Surgery. His research interests are the detection of viral DNA in plasma and peripheral blood mononuclear cells in patients with viral exanthems, the novel applications of digital epiluminescence dermatoscopy and the first applications of regression analyses with bootstrapped simulations to detect epidemics of exanthems. He collaborates with co-investigators from 12 countries, and has published more than 100 articles in journals, books and book chapters. He was honoured at the 14th Congress of the European Academy of Dermatology and Venereology in London as being the principal author of "One of the Most Worth Reading Papers in Medical Dermatology of the Year". He was elected as author of the "Cover Theme Article in Clinical Dermatology of the Year" in *The Yearbook of Dermatology and Dermatologic Surgery 2005*, Mosby. He is an Editor of the *European Journal of Pediatric Dermatology*. He was invited to write a chapter for the *Harper's Textbook of Pediatric Dermatology* which is the bible in paediatric dermatology. He was nominated by Professor Rosie Young for the "Ten Outstanding Young Persons Selection 2006" and was short-listed for the final judging interviews.

❖ Dr. Stephen Kam So **Foo**, MBBS (HK), FHKCFP, FHKAM (Family Medicine), FRACGP (Hon), FAFPM (Hon), FHKCFP (Hon)

Dr. Foo is a family physician in private practice. Graduated from the Medical Faculty of The University of Hong Kong, he worked in the A&E and the Orthopaedic units of Queen Elizabeth Hospital for 3 years. He then served in the Our Lady of Maryknoll Hospital rotating in various clinical disciplines for 2 years before starting his private solo general practice in 1971. In 1977, he was one of the pioneers in establishing the Hong Kong College of General Practitioners (now known as the Hong Kong College of Family Physicians). He has served in the College as a Council Member for the past 30 years and was the President from 1992 to 1998. In 1992, when the Hong Kong Academy of Medicine was established, he was an interim

Council Member of the Academy and was instrumental in making the College a Founding Member of the Academy. He has served in the Academy as a Council Member for 10 years and is now the Honorary Treasurer. He is also the Honorary Clinical Associate Professor in Family Medicine of The University of Hong Kong and the Adjunct Associate Professor in Family Medicine of The Chinese University of Hong Kong.

❖ Dr. Kenny **Kung**, BSc, MBBS, MRCGP, FHKCFP, FRACGP, MFM, FHKAM (Family Medicine), DOM

Dr. Kung is the medical officer-in-charge at the Family Medicine Training Centre, Prince of Wales Hospital, Hong Kong. He graduated from the United Medical and Dental Schools of Guy's and St Thomas' Hospitals in 1999. He has mostly concentrated his research on current primary care practice at a local level, with its impact on the population and on frontline doctors. Since initiating research in 2003, he has published and presented over 15 articles in both local journals and overseas conferences.

❖ Dr. Augustine Tsan **Lam**, MB, BS (HKU), FRACGP, FHKCFP, FHKAM (Family Medicine)

Dr. Lam is the Chief of Service of the Department of Family Medicine, New Territories East Cluster, Hospital Authority, HKSAR, China. He is also the adjunct Associate Professor in the Department of Community and Family Medicine at The Chinese University of Hong Kong.

He graduated from The University of Hong Kong in 1985 and received training in Hong Kong. He has extensive clinical experience working in local family practice settings. His main interests are in the Vocational Training Programme in Family Medicine and future development of the specialty of family medicine in Hong Kong and China. He works closely with the faculty of medicine of two local universities in undergraduate teaching and conducting numerous researches related to family practice and clinical audits.

❖ Professor Philip Kam-Tao **Li**, MBBS, MD, MRCP, FRCP (Lond, Edin), FACP, FHKCP, FHKAM (Medicine)

Professor Li is the Director of the Family Medicine Training Centre in the Prince of Wales Hospital, Hong Kong. He is also the Chief of Nephrology and Consultant Physician of the Department of Medicine and Therapeutics at the Prince of Wales Hospital. He is the Honorary Professor of Medicine at The Chinese University of Hong Kong and the Deputy Hospital Chief Executive of the Prince of Wales Hospital.

He is the past Chairman of the Hong Kong Society of Nephrology. Currently he is the Council Member of the International Society of Nephrology (ISN) as well as of the Asian Pacific Society of Nephrology. He is also the Vice President of the Hong Kong Transplantation Society. He also serves as the Honorary Secretary at the Hong Kong College of Physicians.

Professor Li is the founding Editor-in-Chief of the *Hong Kong Journal of Nephrology*, Deputy Editor of *Nephrology* and Editor of the *Nephrology Dialysis and Transplantation* and *International Journal of Artificial Organs*. He is on the Editorial Boards of *Peritoneal Dialysis International, Chinese Journal of Nephrology, Dialysis & Transplantation* and *Medical Progress*. He is a regular reviewer for all the major nephrology journals and many general medical journals.

He has published over 300 original and review articles in peer-reviewed journals, 2 books and 13 book chapters. He has been invited as a speaker at over 50 international congresses and meetings.

His research interests include prevention of progression of chronic kidney disease, IgA nephropathy, diabetes in renal failure and immunogenetics of nephropathies, peritoneal dialysis and cardiovascular mortality in dialysis patients.

❖ Dr. Donald Kwok Tung **Li**

Dr. Li is a specialist in family medicine in private practice. He was President of the Hong Kong College of Family Physicians, a position he held from 1998 to 2004.

Dr. Li graduated with his first degree (BA) from Cornell University, USA, followed by his second degree (MBBS) from The University of Hong Kong, in 1975 and 1980 respectively. He is an Honorary Fellow of the Hong Kong College of Family Physicians, Honorary Fellow of the Royal Australian College of General Practitioners, Honorary Fellow of the Hong Kong College of Dental Surgeons and Fellow of the Hong Kong Academy of Medicine. Dr. Li holds a number of other distinguished professional memberships, including Honorary Secretary of the Past President's Advisory Committee of the Hong Kong Academy of Medicine and is the newly elected President of WONCA Asia Pacific Region for 2007–2009.

He is an active member of many Hong Kong governmental and public health bodies. He also dedicates much of his professional time to academia and teaching, including as Member of Council of Cornell University; Honorary Assistant Professor in the Faculty of Medicine, The University of Hong Kong; Honorary Adjunct Associate Professor in Family Medicine at The Chinese University of Hong Kong; Honorary Consultant at Huashan Hospital, Shanghai, China; and Lecturer of the Diploma of Family Medicine of the Hong Kong College of Family Physicians as well as examiner of the conjoint RACGP/HKCFP Fellowship Examination. Dr. Li has been a member of the Ethic's Committee of the Medical Council of Hong Kong since 1996. He is also a member of the Board of Directors of the Hospital Authority which governs all the public hospitals in Hong Kong.

Dr. Li is Director of the Bauhinia Research Foundation, a civic think-tank. He is also a member of the Board of Stewards of the Hong Kong Jockey Club, one of the biggest charitable funding organisations in Hong Kong. Dr. Li also serves on the council of the St. John's Ambulance of Hong Kong.

Dr. Li has been an invited speaker at numerous local, regional and international scientific meetings. Throughout his career, he has been a leading expert and ardent advocate in promoting better primary care and family health in Hong Kong and the region.

❖ Dr. Christopher **Tong**, MBChB (Hons), FRCSEd, FCSHK, FHKCOS, FRCSEd (Orth), FHKAM (Orthopaedic Surgery)

Dr. Tong graduated from the University of Edinburgh in 1994 (MBChB [Hons]). He subsequently completed his orthopaedic specialist training in Hong Kong in 2001. He is currently in private practice in Hong Kong specialising in orthopaedic surgery. His main clinical interests include knee and shoulder surgery and sports medicine. He is Honorary Sports Medicine Consultant at the Hong Kong Sports Institute and also Honorary Clinical Assistant Professor at The Chinese University of Hong Kong.

❖ Dr. Clement K. K. **Tsang**

Dr. Tsang is currently the Professor of Institute of Hospital Administration, Ministry of Health, China and Deputy Director of Research and Development Centre for General Practice, Ministry of Health, China.

❖ Dr. **Wong** Hung Wai, MBBS (HK), FRCGP, FRACGP, FHKAM (Family Medicine), FHKCFP, DFM (CUHK), DCH (Lond)

Dr. Wong is a Family Medicine specialist in private practice. He graduated from The University of Hong Kong in 1975. He has vast experience in Training and Assessment, having been the Chairman of the Board of Examination of the Hong Kong College of Family Physicians from 1997 to 2004. He worked as a part-time Consultant in Family Medicine for the Hospital Authority from 2000 to 2005. He is still a Family Medicine trainer for both Basic and Higher trainees of the College of Family Physicians. He now has great interest in dermatology including cosmetic procedures.

❖ Professor Samuel Yeung Shan **Wong**, MD (University of Toronto), CCFP, FRCACGP

Professor Wong received his doctor of medicine degree from the University of Toronto and completed his residency training in Family Medicine at Dalhousie University, Canada. He is a certificate member of the Canadian College of Family Practice and a Fellow of the Royal Australian College of General Practitioners. His main research interests are mind and body medicine, mental health in the community and primary care, men's health and male osteoporosis. His funded research work included a randomised controlled trial study of the effectiveness of mind-body intervention on chronic pain, studies investigating the comorbidity of depressive illnesses with major medical conditions and psychological and genitourinary problems facing Hong Kong middle-aged and elderly males. The results of his research were disseminated to the general public through 34 newspaper reports and 3 TV interviews.

❖ Dr. William Po Tin **Yip**, MBBS (HK), FRCS (G), FHKCORL, FHKAM (Specialist in ORL)

Dr. Yip graduated from The University of Hong Kong in 1965. After internship he received general surgical training in the Professorial Surgical Unit, The University of Hong Kong.

In 1968 Dr. Yip went to the UK for postgraduate training in Otorhinolaryngology. Having worked in the Royal National Throat, Nose and Ear Hospital and several Hospitals in the UK, Dr. Yip was appointed Consultant ENT surgeon in the Edgware General Hospital and the Whittington Hospital in North London from 1979 till 1982. On returning to

Hong Kong in 1982 Dr. Yip set up his own private clinic in Central till now.

Dr. Yip was elected Foundation Fellow of both the College of Otorhinolaryngology of Hong Kong and the Academy of Medicine of Hong Kong in 1994. He was also President of the Society of Otorhinolaryngolgy, Head and Neck Surgery of Hong Kong from 1993 to 1997.

Dr. Yip is the Honorary Clinical Associate Professor in ENT at both The University of Hong Kong and The Chinese University of Hong Kong, participating in active clinical teaching of the undergraduates of both universities. He is also the Honorary ENT Consultant in the Hong Kong Sanatorium & Hospital.

❖ Dr. **Yiu** Yuk Kwan, MBBS (HKU), DCH (Irel), Dip Practical Dermatology (Wales), FHKCP, FRACGP, FHKAM (Family Medicine)

Dr. Yiu is the Chief of Service of the Department of Family Medicine and Primary Health Care, Kowloon West Cluster, Hospital Authority, HKSAR, China. She graduated from the University of Hong Kong in 1989 and was amongst the earliest batch Family Medicine trainee in Hong Kong. She completed her basic training in Evangel Hospital, one of the major pioneer private hospitals dedicated to Family Medicine training in Hong Kong. She then joined the Hospital Authority to pursue her career and devoted most of her time to the FM development in the Hospital Authority as well as in Hong Kong. Her main interest is Family Medicine Training and she dedicated most of her time to developing high quality training for FM doctors in Hospital Authority and she has been working closely with the Hong Kong College of Family Physician. She is interested in teaching and was adjunct Associate Professor of the Department of Community and Family Medicine at The Chinese University of Hong Kong.

❖ Professor Nat **Yuen**, MB.BS (QLD), MD (HON, QLD), MICGP, FRACGP, FHCFP, HKAM (Family Medicine), DTM&H (SYD), DFM (CUHK)

Professor Yuen graduated with a degree in Medicine from the University of Queensland, Australia, 1965. He was awarded Honorary Doctor of Medicine by the University of Queensland in 1995, and Honorary Fellow of the Royal Australian College of General Practitioners in 2004. Professor Yuen has a long record in community service. He was the President of the

Hong Kong Medical Association, President of the Hong Kong College of General Practitioners, Chairman of the Medical and Health Development Advisory Committee of Hong Kong, and in the past few years, he has been appointed as Honorary Clinical Professor of Family Medicine of The Chinese University of Hong Kong and Censor-in-Chief of the Hong Kong College of Family Physicians. His publications include *Principles and Practice of Primary Care and Family Medicine, Asia-Pacific Perspectives*, edited by John Fry and Nat Yuen, 1994, and many articles in *JAMA SEA* and *Journal of the Hong Kong College of General Practitioners*.

SECTION I

Principles of Diagnosis and Management

Chapter 1

Consultation Skills

◆ WONG Hung Wai ◆

> The generalist cannot take refuge in the limitations of his specialty. For him the healing relationship must be entered in the fullest sense ... He must help, care for, comfort and ease when the specialist has nothing to offer ... The patient often has made the rounds of the specialties; he is still ill, still needing answers to the key clinical questions. Even if the patient's illness has been "negotiated" out of medicine by other physicians, someone must remain who can help. The generalist, on this view, is the physician par excellence since he has the most intimate relationship with the healing and helping functions of medicine. A specialist, especially if his domain is a technique, might get away with only scientifically right decisions; but a generalist, never.
>
> (Pellegrino 1983, "The Healing Relationship", in Shelp (ed.) *The Clinical Encounter.* Dordrecht: D. Reidel, p. 166.)

To appreciate how family doctors work, you need to have some understanding of what they do and of the differences between them and their secondary care colleagues.

What is a family doctor?

The family doctor's role cannot be defined in a single phrase. Just like the family doctor's approach to patients, it is defined in a holistic way.

The following definition (or more accurately description) is based upon that given by the Royal College of General Practitioners (UK), The Royal Australian College of General Practitioners, the American Academy of Family Physicians and The College of Family Physicians of Canada. Some discrepancies exist among the professional bodies due to cultural needs and differing health systems, but some essential elements can be seen:

Primary care

- Family doctors are the point of first contact for a defined population
- They provide comprehensive health care encompassing the physical, psychological and social aspects of early diagnosis, and initial and continuing management of acute, chronic and terminal problems in patients and their families
- They provide treatment, prevention and education for promoting health care for patients, families and the community
- They tend to be patient-centred, including understanding the impact illnesses have on patients and their families and empowering and collaborating with patients as partners, thus creating a unique doctor-patient-family relationship

Specialist care

- Specialists are trained with in-depth knowledge or skills in one particular area of medicine
- They may be skilled at dealing with ambiguity and uncertainty
- They should work closely with other primary care team members to achieve optimal care for the sick
- They should be aware of their strengths and recognise their limitations, especially following the Bristol case in the UK (Dyer 2001)

Other roles of a family doctor

Stewardship

Family doctors have the social responsibility of helping to manage limited resources whilst weighing up the needs of the individual against those of the community

Advocacy

At the community level, family doctors should advocate both the health of individual patients and also the interests of the general public

In 1994, the WONCA (World Organization of National Colleges, Academies and Academic Associations) and WHO convened a meeting and recommended that doctors should have a central role in the achievement of quality, cost effectiveness and equity in health care systems.

Differences between family and hospital-based doctors

To understand how a family doctor makes a diagnosis, one has to acknowledge the different circumstances in which a hospital doctor works. Once this becomes apparent, it is clear that family doctors do not have the time (or the need) to go through the same history-taking procedure as that of a hospital doctor. Some of the obvious differences are listed below:

- Family doctors usually see a new patient every 5–15 minutes (some have and some do not have appointments, but nevertheless the time span for seeing patients is more or less the same) (see "Appointment systems—opening the door to better access?", http://www.innovate .org.uk/library/DoncasterAccess/Doncasterreport.htm).

- Due to ease of access (by virtue of close vicinity to patients and flexibility of appointment), family doctors can be far more adaptable as to when and how often they wish to review the patient. This also allows the patient to be reviewed according to their illness and need instead of appointment availability.

- Family doctors usually work in the same practice and community for many years. This gives an opportunity to provide continuity of care to an individual and often to the other family members too. Consequently, the family doctor gets to know the patient both medically and quasi-socially ("quasi" as the knowledge of their patient is an accumulation over time of what the patient or family members tell them, and possibly from having seen the patient in their home during home visits). With the current increase in group practices, it is important that continuity of information (as a form of continuity of care) be maintained.

- A family doctor is trained as a generalist. They need to know about most common ailments in respect to their epidemiology so that they can guide the patient as to whether or not the treatment being received from secondary care is appropriate, thus acting as the patient's personal advisor and advocate.

- Access to investigations is variable depending on the place of practice.

However family doctors are trained to work with limited resources and do not always need the more complex investigations. In certain circumstances, their role is to identify those patients who need further investigations or treatment, e.g. in the case of a malignancy, and to refer to the specialist for further management.

• Due to lack of immediacy of investigation, a family doctor has to live with ambiguity and the fact that most diagnoses are made on probability based on history, examination and sometimes trial of treatment.

• The presentation can be covert. That is to say that the patient presents with one issue but really comes to see the doctor for another problem which they are far more concerned about but has difficulty in talking about, such as mental health issues and sexual problems. The family doctor thus has to try to recognise this type of scenario and to elucidate the real reason for the attendance.

• A family doctor can act as a gatekeeper to control access to secondary care. However this role is largely dependent on the type of healthcare system. In places such as Hong Kong and the US, patients can have access to specialists in the private sector directly. On the other hand, patients in the British National Health Service would have to go through their family doctor or Accident and Emergency department first for their secondary care referral.

In one type of US model, the patient accesses a multi-specialty primary care centre in which both family doctors and other specialty-trained doctors, together with specially-trained nurses and non-medical staff, may see and treat the patients (Feachem 2002). Interestingly, Forrest (2003) asserts that the gatekeeper role is not the cause of, but a reflection of, lower healthcare spending/resources in a country. However it does lead to fewer unsuitable patients being seen by the specialists and a reduction in inappropriate investigations and management of patients. Furthermore, most patients appreciate the role of a family doctor in helping them to work out and to match their needs with currently available resources.

The importance of the consultation

Most of the work of a family doctor is carried out inside the consultation room. Such patient-doctor encounters are the cornerstone of the care delivered to the family doctor's patients, including life-saving incidents, simple advice on diet, life habits, prevention of disease, management of minor, self-limiting problems, management of long-standing chronic conditions, and many others. Failure to carry out an efficient and effective consultation affects the outcome of patient care unfavourably. Hence it is desirable to develop high competence in consultation skills. We will concentrate on the tasks of the consultation using a task-orientated model—what makes the consultation fail and how to improve consultation skills.

Consultation models

Consultation models can best be described as "what doctors do in the consultation and how they do it". Many books have and will continue to be written about how doctors carry out the consultation process. However most books are written for postgraduate doctors. There is really no reason for this other than that many educationalists feel (as do most students) that there is so much to learn, so why burden students with more.

The alternative view would be that if you gain some understanding now as to how a consultation process evolves or is conducted, then you are less likely to make the same errors as your current tutors did!

What we propose here is to give you a brief summary as to the main types of consultation processes so that you may gain some ideas.

Doctor-centred approach

According to Phase II of the Byrne and Long model, it is the doctor who is responsible for discovering the reason(s) for the patient's attendance (Byrne and Long 1976). Invariably, the doctor will guide the patient in order to obtain the information they regard as useful and discard other information, and will process this information to fit their health system and do what they think is the best for the patient. For example, "I need to make a diagnosis to sort out this problem. The first task is to take a history ..." and so forth. This may also lead to performing other tasks such as reminding the patient about lifestyle changes they need to make generally in order to remain well, dealing with pre-existing diseases, or advising them how to access healthcare services more appropriately.

Patient-centred approach

In this approach the doctor will try to find out in what way and how the patient sees the change in his/her mind or body. This is particularly useful when resistance is felt to the doctor's recommendation, or patients fail to comply, or there is no improvement despite changes in management. However the downside of this approach is that the doctor may need to spend a lot of time with a particular patient to explore the hidden agenda, either at the expense of other patients or indeed their own well-being. Sometimes there may be an undesirable effect on patients who merely want some symptomatic relief for the common cold or who are used to a doctor-centred approach, leading to conflicts or mistrust in the relationship.

Behaviour-orientated approach

This best describes how the doctor conducts the interview itself. Either by working with the patient to solve the problem or, at the other end of the spectrum, assuming they know what the patient wants or needs without even asking. A good example of the latter is how medical professionals often write in the consultation notes: "Patient Reassured" after a particular diagnosis is made. Nowhere in the notes is it written (for it is never asked) what exactly it is that the patient is most worried about!

The reality is that we all use all these various approaches all the time, but vary our style according to the patient, the situation and how we are feeling at the time.

Tasks

In the normal run of events, the family doctor may want to achieve the following:

- Identify the reasons for consultation
- Define the problem
- Address the problem
- Explain the problem to the patient
- Make effective use of the consultation

Identifying the reasons for consultation

The importance of this cannot be over-emphasised, yet it is often overlooked. This may be due to limit of tolerance, limit of anxiety, presenting with a trivial or unrelated problem masking the actual problem (hidden agenda) or the actual patient presenting as an accompanying person, or administrative reasons (McWhinney 1997). A patient with chest pain may come to see you because the pain is so severe that they cannot tolerate it. They may also come because they are worried that they may have something wrong with their heart. A young mother may bring her perfectly normal first-born baby to see you repeatedly for minor complaints, but actually she is the one requiring help as she is not coping well in taking care of the baby. A patient may also come for administrative reasons such as a pre-employment checkup or a sick leave certificate.

Defining the problem

Information required for defining the problem is gathered by history taking, appropriate physical examination and simple surgery tests. It is necessary to establish the effects of the illness on work and everyday social life, taking into consideration physical, psychological, social and financial factors. Is the patient able to go to school or work as usual? Is sleep affected? Then explore the patient's own interpretation of the problem; their ideas, concerns and expectations. Are they worried about some severe condition like cancer? How do they think the doctor can help them?

The next stage in defining the problem is making a working diagnosis. In primary care, detailed clinical diagnoses are uncommon. Patients often present with problems at an early stage which are unspecific and undifferentiated in nature and lack the features required to make a definitive diagnosis. A working diagnosis is one on which the doctor can formulate further plans for refinement of the diagnosis as the condition progresses or changes, or on which a management plan is based.

Addressing the problem

How severe is the problem? Is it life-threatening and warrants immediate referral? The four main conditions a family doctor cannot afford to miss are coronary heart disease, severe infections, cancers and ectopic pregnancy (Murtagh 1998), although cerebrovascular accidents should be added to this list due to recent advances in its management.

If urgent referral is not required, the doctor will formulate a management plan appropriate to the working diagnosis, involving the patient in the decision-making process. The patient should be told about all available options and the pros and cons of each before choices are made. This way the risk of disagreement and litigation will be much less.

Explaining the problem to the patient

This is essential but is often neglected or done in a half-hearted way. If a specific clinical condition is diagnosed, its possible causes, course, available treatments and possible side-effects, and prognosis should be clearly explained. Warn the patient that the condition may change and, if certain signs or symptoms appear, a different course of action may be required. The doctor should not use medical jargon, and the language and manner should be appropriate to the patient's background and linked to their health beliefs. Throughout the process the doctor needs to demonstrate that they are honest and sympathetic as well as empathetic. Try to strike a balance among priorities with the patient—not always an easy task. Keep checking with the patient that they understand you.

Making effective use of the consultation

There are three components to this: making efficient use of available resources, establishing an effective relationship with the patient and giving opportunistic health promotion advice.

Resources include time, investigations, other health professionals and medications. Time management is obviously important for the busy doctor. What matters is the way the time is spent with the patient, not just the length of time. Any investigation ordered must help in confirming or excluding the working diagnosis, or in follow-up consultations, and contribute to the monitoring of the treatment of the patient. Costs should also be considered. Investigations done just to reassure the patient can rarely be justified. Other health professionals such as physiotherapists and dietitians are members of the primary health care team and the family doctor maintains overall responsibility even when they are involved in patient management. Medication should only be given when strictly necessary and accompanied by all explanations and precautions.

There is no single best way to build an effective relationship with the patient. Different doctors use different ways. An efficient patient-doctor relationship facilitates successful completion of the tasks of the consultation. Most important in this relationship is the element of trust. To achieve this, good communication skills are essential.

Since the family doctor sees a large number of patients every day, the impact regarding prevention in the long run can be enormous. Opportunistic health promotion should be an integral part of all primary care consultations, be it anti-smoking advice, exercise advice, blood pressure measurement, fall prevention in the elderly or checking pap smear screening in women.

Why a consultation fails

There are many reasons why a consultation will not result in the desired outcome. The following are some of the reasons and the possible solutions:

- Inadequate preparation by the doctor—review patient's record beforehand, get to know the patient by name, their background, medical history, etc.
- Failure to prepare the patient, long waiting time—clinic protocol to inform patient of the explanation
- Premature interruptions, not allowing the patient to finish their opening statement—let patient tell the story in their own words, with adequate time
- Restricted focus, assuming patient has only one problem—be aware that patients have an average of three to four problems; also, organic and psychosocial problems often co-exist
- Failure to detect inconsistencies in the patient's history—attempt to clarify with the patient any doubts about the accuracy of understanding of the history
- Failure to respond to verbal and non-verbal cues, especially of emotional origin—listen to the patient carefully, maintain good eye contact, do not be too occupied with writing notes or with the keyboard
- Using too many closed-ended direct questions—use open-ended questioning especially at the early stages of the interview, allow ample time for the patient to explain
- Giving too much information and advice to the patient at one consultation—be realistic, do not expect the patient to remember everything; use written instructions and pamphlets to help

How to improve consultation skills?

To consult effectively and efficiently one must have a genuine liking for people and be warm, caring and conscientious. Good communication skills are a must for successful consulting. To start with there are a few basic things to remember:

- The patient sitting in front of you is a person, not a "case"
- Every patient is unique, with their own health beliefs, illness behaviours and cultural background.

- Patient welfare is the top priority; in other words, always think about what is best for the patient

- The single most important thing that affects the outcome of the consultation is the patient-doctor relationship—put simply, the patient's trust in you

- Most of the time, a patient-centred approach is more desirable than a doctor-centred approach

Summary

Communication skills are now part of the undergraduate medical curriculum; vocational training programmes and diploma courses in family medicine all put emphasis on this aspect. Problems with doctor-patient communication are extremely common and adversely affect patient management. It has been repeatedly shown that the clinical skills needed to improve these problems can be taught and that the subsequent benefits to medical practice are demonstrable and enduring.

References

Byrne, P. S. and Long, B. E. L. 1976. *Doctors Talking to Patients. Another carefully researched and pioneering study of doctors' verbal behavioral.* London: HMSO.

Dyer, C. 2001. "Bristol inquiry condemns hospital's 'club culture'". *British Medical Journal*, 323 (7306): 181.

Feachem, R. G. A. 2002. "Commission on macroeconomics and health". *Bulletin of the World Health Organization,* 80 (2): 87.

Forrest, C. B. 2003. "Primary care in the United States: Primary care gatekeeping and referrals: Effective filter or failed experiment?". *British Medical Journal,* 326 (7391): 692–695.

Murtagh, J. 1998. *General Practice* (2nd edition). Sydney: McGraw-Hill.

McWhinney, I. R. 1997. *A Textbook of Family Medicine* (2nd edition). New York: Oxford University Press.

Shelp, E. E. (ed.). 1983. *The Clinical Encounter: The Moral Fabric of the Patient-Physician Relationship.* Dordrecht: D. Reidel Publishing Company.

Chapter 2

Diagnosis in Primary Care

◆ Martin LINDSAY ◆

How to be a "good doctor" whilst making it easier to form a diagnosis

It is said that 56–83% of diagnoses are made on history alone (Hamptons 1975; Sadler 1979). Here are the clues:

There are four essentials for any good doctor:

"Listen, listen further, listen some more, <u>then</u> talk."

Listen

By giving patients time to talk.

 Many a diagnosis is missed by not allowing patients enough time to talk. Active listening saves thousands of words.

Your approach should always be welcoming. Greet the patient—perhaps, if time allows and especially if you have not met previously, have a chat about something unrelated to why they are coming to see you. This helps enormously in relaxing the patient, makes them feel they are being treated in a caring manner and that they are important, and that you, as the professional, are quite at ease in talking to anyone (remember many patients prefer nurses to doctors as doctors are perceived to be snobbish and too busy to understand their patients) (Horrocks et al. 2002). This then helps to break down barriers and, especially in primary care, makes it more likely that they feel they are able to address sensitive areas such as sexual or mental health problems.

Listen

By giving non-verbal cues.

 Appear relaxed. Nod and use other non-verbal methods to indicate that you are attentive to and interested in what the patient is saying.

Ideally the room should be welcoming wherever possible. Obviously this is not always possible in a hospital setting. However if you do have any influence, try to ensure that you have a comfortable chair for the patient (preferably the same size as yours). Have some pleasant pictures on the wall. Hide those wall charts of the half-dissected human body. Damien Hirst won the Turner prize (a leading British Arts award) with his "Mother and Child Divided" in 1995 (the one with the cow cut in half, fixed in formalin and placed in a glass cabinet), and no doubt many people found his piece of art wonderful, but how many of us really want to see something similar when we go to the doctor about our own body?

Think about the relative positions of yourself, the patient and the desk. Sitting behind a desk separates you from the patient both physically and psychologically—something then comes between you and the patient, again both physically but also emotionally. Try, for example, to sit on the same side of the table or just across a corner of the table. Not only does this help eliminate the hierarchy of parent-child relationship but you can also see the patient's body language more easily (and they you—so be careful).

Be aware of your own body and hand gestures, the tone, speed, pitch and volume of your voice, and your movements and facial expressions. People who make direct eye contact when talking are often perceived as strong, honest and straightforward. Dane Archer, a Professor at the University of California at Santa Cruz, has produced videotapes on this subject. They can be accessed on http://nonverbal.ucsc.edu/. Other useful sites include The Center for Non Verbal Studies at http://members.aol.com/nonverbal2.

Personality has an effect on vocal behaviour as well as on pitch, breathlessness (volume and rate), vocal cues and variety (Masterson 1996). Also, in speaking, both language (verbal aspects or words) and paralanguage (vocal aspects or sounds) play significant roles in conveying our meaning (Buchholz 1998).

Listen

By allowing time.

 Appear unhurried. Give the patient time to convey not only the history but also their concerns.

The following are some of the techniques you may use:

Echoing: To ensure you have understood the patient and that the patient is aware that you have understood them, repeat the problem/history back to the patient. This encourages the patient to tell you more of the history.

Summarising: Summarise the points that have been covered. This helps to ensure mutual understanding and agreement. It can be used when a large number of topics are being covered, especially with elderly people, or to gather thoughts when stuck. It also helps to buy time and think through complex issues.

Clarifying: As the word implies, it is used when the illness experience described by the patient becomes unclear or irrational. Sometimes it helps you to see from the patient's point of view and at other times it helps the patient to verbalise their beliefs.

Reflecting: This is a step beyond clarifying and is commonly used to help patients to gain more insight into their "irrational" beliefs or behaviour.

Challenging: This can be used in restricting attitude or behaviour; or to give direct feedback within a caring context.

Talk

Explain the diagnosis, investigations required, and proposed management including the drugs (if any) and their side-effects. Always try to imagine what the problem must feel like from the patient's perspective. By doing this you might be able to answer many of their concerns without them either asking or indeed realising what their concerns are at the time of the consultation.

Empower the patient: let them be an equal partner in the decision-making process. Explain how you see the problem and its solution. Encourage the patient to ask questions, no matter how stupid, puerile or naive these may appear. It is often these "silly" questions that allow them to begin to comprehend both the problem and its solution. As some people would say, "The only really dumb question is the one you take home with you."

Discuss the prognosis and outcome with the patient. What should happen if all goes well and what might happen if it does not. If it does not, what should the patient do and what will you do? This also serves to allay the patient's fear, for if you have thought about what might go wrong so have they!

Above all, always use simple words and phrases. When students first enter medicine they speak the same simple language as everyone else. By the time they are qualified their language has become so corrupted by jargon that any non-medical person would have difficulty understanding what they are talking about. They then spend the next decade or more in postgraduate courses trying to re-learn how the rest of civilisation speaks!

As George Orwell once stated:

- Never use a long word where a short one will do
- If it is possible to cut a word out, always cut it out
- Never use the passive where you can use the active
- Never use a foreign phrase, a scientific word or a jargon if you can think of an everyday equivalent

Diagnosis in family medicine

Ultimately, the main reason any patient comes to see the doctor is for a diagnosis to be made and a cure to be offered. Many, if not most, will accept that treatment per se even though it may not always be necessary due to the self-limiting nature of many illnesses. The diagnostic process needs to take into account not only the history of the complaint and examination of the patient, but also the psychosocial aspects of that person too.

Difficulties for family doctors

So, despite the above advice, why do family doctors sometimes miss a diagnosis on initial presentation?

1. *Diseases presented at an early level or stage are not always immediately recognisable*

For example, shingles. The patient comes complaining of itchy skin. The rash may only appear one week after the start of the symptoms. If the patient presents in the intervening time only dry skin will be seen (as is often the case as shingles tends to be an illness of the elderly who often have dry skin as part of the aging process). More recently, patients with SARS were missed due to their atypical presentations (Tomlinson and Cockram 2003).

2. *Language difficulties/Ethnic minorities*

Patients whose first tongue is not that of the local language will have difficulty in communicating. Interpreters can be used, but the standard can fluctuate enormously between the most basic (e.g. the 5-year-old son translating about his mother's gynaecological problem) to the level of professional interpreters. There are also innovative telephone translation services. However no matter who does the translating there is always some loss of meaning, which may be even more relevant in mental health issues.

It is recognised that people from different cultures may talk about and present their illnesses in different ways. Europeans, for example, may come complaining of a sore throat, aches and pains, and a headache. Clearly the diagnosis is an upper respiratory tract infection. An African may, on the other hand, talk mostly about feeling weak and having painful joints, and omit to say anything about the sore throat.

3. *Cultural/Belief patterns*

Greenhalgh et al. found that health beliefs and folk models of diabetes in British Bangladeshis had both many similarities and differences in body image, cause and nature of diabetes, and knowledge of complications (Greenhalgh et al. 1998). Asthmatic patients of South Asian and white racial background differed in their confidence in their family doctors and utilisation of the service, as shown in a qualitative study by Griffiths et al. (2001).

Just as important, the doctors' own belief patterns can cause prejudice in a consultation, e.g. a patient expecting to receive antibiotics for URTI is three times more likely to get it whereas a doctor perceiving their patient wanting antibiotics would result in a ten-fold increase of prescription (Cockburn and Pit 1997). Furthermore, tools developed for the West may not be applicable in other racial or cultural settings, e.g. there are substantial variations in the rates of detection of anxiety and depressive symptoms in primary care patients using General Health Questionnaire-12. Such symptoms may be under-diagnosed in Asian patients in particular (Comino et al. 2001).

4. *Covert presentation*

The commonest example would be a patient who presents with multiple problems. They then only mention the most serious problem briefly among the verbosity of their other complaints.

5. *Age-related*

It is well recognised that the same disease can be presented differently according to the patient's age. The elderly, for example, do not always present with a cough and pyrexia when they have a severe chest infection, but will only mention lethargy or being generally unwell.

6. *Own emotions*

The doctor may be uneasy at dealing with the patient's emotions and hence their verbal and/or non-verbal cues suggest that the patient change the subject. Similarly, the doctor may say or do something inadvertently that the patient feels uneasy about. This then inhibits conversation from the patient. Lack of detachment by the doctor can occasionally occur. This would affect the way a doctor looks at the situation and their objectivity.

7. *Fear and over-reaction*

The doctor's fear (whether about litigation or related to adverse past experience) can lead to over-investigation and/or referral. Sometimes it may simply be related to job stress in general. Therefore a competent doctor should be able to recognise their own mounting stress level and be prepared to do something constructive about it.

8. *The consulting environment*

This can have a major bearing—if the room is not properly laid out or there are continued interruptions. With the increased use of computers the computer can become the centre of attention and not the patient!

9. *Frequent attendees/"Heart-sink" patients*

Just like "the boy who cried wolf", it is so easy to miss something serious. Physical illnesses tend to be missed in mental patients (Phelan 2001). Good management techniques are needed to curb these patients—probably the best method is to try to understand and determine why they need to see the doctor so often (i.e. their underlying necessity and motive) and to deal with that underlying reason for attending.

The diagnostic pathway

This overview shows the process by which family doctors come to a conclusion as to how to treat or manage the situation. Note that the term diagnosis is deliberately not used, as sometimes a definite conclusion cannot be reached (see below). Also be aware that some of the headings used are more for clarification rather than as a term of acceptance in their own right.

- "**Which Method**" is used to make a diagnosis based on history alone
- The **Provisional Diagnosis** is then reached (based solely on the history)
- **Examination** is undertaken to reach a more selected group of diagnoses (Pre-test Probable Diagnosis)
- **Investigations** are decided upon history and examination
- Patient reviewed with the test results (**Post-test Probable Diagnosis**)

The all too common outcomes:

- A **Working Diagnosis** is not an unusual outcome
- **Managing Uncertainty** is often a reality

The four methods of making a diagnosis

It is recognised that there are four broad ways in which a diagnosis is made in medicine:

1. *Pattern recognition*

For example, Parkinson's disease (as the patient shuffles in with a plain expression on their face and tremulous hands).

It is obvious that to solely use this method presupposes not only an extensive knowledge base for every single disease (impossible to attain) but also that many diseases have the same/similar pattern of presentation.

2. *Algorithm*

This can best be described as a step-by-step approach for reaching a clinical decision or diagnosis. It is often set out in the form of a flow chart, in which the answer to each question determines the next question to be asked. It is similar to computerised management protocols used in nursing triage systems (Richards et al. 2002) or management guidelines for diagnosis of hypertension produced by British Hypertension Society

(Williams et al. 2004). Whilst very helpful in standardising diagnosing criteria for certain conditions, it only covers a limited number of conditions and, more importantly, does not take account of individual circumstances.

3. *Inductive method*

This is the time-honoured approach by all students (yes, including the authors) of taking an in-depth, systematic history followed by a full examination of all systems. It is often the first diagnostic method introduced to medical students and is designed mainly for hospital use when the doctors have had no previous contact with the patient or the patient's problems cannot be resolved by the generalists. It is used by even the most experienced clinician when unsure of what the problem is or what to do next!

The effectiveness of this approach is largely unknown and is regarded as "unhelpful advice from textbooks" by some (Del and Glasziou 2003). Whether it is based on ritual or evidence, this method is an exhaustive process and would take too long in a primary care setting if done for every case.

4. *Hypothetico-deductive method*

Unlike the inductive method, when only facts are used to make a diagnosis, this method makes an assumption and then the facts are sought, i.e. it works in reverse to the inductive method (McWhinney 1989).

Put more practically, a hypothetical diagnosis is made (i.e. what is the most common and therefore likely cause) and the doctor looks at what facts can be used to confirm or refute this possibility. In reality there are usually two or three possible diagnoses at any one time.

As a simple example—a middle-aged, overweight man who smokes comes in to see you complaining of chest pain. The first thoughts you, the family doctor, would (or should) have are "Is this angina? Or gastro-oesophageal reflux or anterior chest wall pains? These are still going to be the most likely causes so let's ask specific questions about these particular illnesses." The reality is that in most cases your hypothetical diagnosis would be correct (simply based on the epidemiology of the disease) but if it is not, at least you have excluded some important causes.

In the following section, we will guide you through a number of examples in detail and show you how the hypothetico-deductive method is used in a clinical setting.

How do family doctors work?

Based on the hypothetico-deductive method, diagnoses can be divided into three categories:

1. The most likely diagnoses (based on probability)
2. The important diagnoses (those that are less likely statistically but must not be missed due to seriousness or because they are eminently treatable)
3. "Novelty" diagnoses (those rare possibilities which clinicians love to remember, often at the expense of those common problems!)

Provisional diagnosis

Usually at the end of the hypothetico-deductive process, a *provisional diagnosis* should have been made. It has been reached based on the terms of probability.

Pre-test probable diagnosis

The examination, which then occurs, should help to confirm or refute some or all of the provisional diagnoses and lead to what could be termed a *pre-test probability* of the disease(s). Investigations can now be requested to help confirm or refute suspicions.

Post-test probable diagnosis

The patient is then reviewed in the light of those results and management implemented based on the *post-test probability* of the disease. Sometimes, however, it is still not always possible to make a definite diagnosis. Sandler (1979) found that no firm diagnosis was made in around 27% of cases after history, examination and investigations in a medical outpatient setting, and such uncertainty could be even higher in a primary care setting.

What next then?

After a working diagnosis is made, we then review the patient or act based on a combination of seriousness (such as one of the four most sinister scenarios: cancer, serious infection, coronary heart disease or ectopic pregnancy) and the patient's circumstances and wishes. Sometimes a diagnosis is all the patient wants. In other cases "watch and see" or "masterly inactivity" may give you time to determine your next course of action. Family doctors have the advantage in that they provide continuing care to their patients and so can monitor the condition closely.

Sometimes one would use the concept of *non-disease diagnosis*, e.g. non-cardiac chest pain, non-specific joint pain. As the prevalence rates of serious illnesses with obvious physical signs at the early stage are very low in primary care, the positive predictive value for diagnostic procedures will be low. Using the non-disease approach will increase the pre-test probability to facilitate the diagnostic process. In primary care it is more important to rule out illnesses with serious consequences.

Alternatively, medication is started either for symptomatic or partially diagnostic purposes. "Is this cough a variant of asthma?" A trial of a beta-antagonist such as salbutamol may be diagnostic in itself. Another example would be a trial of a simple antacid and lifestyle adjustment for new dyspepsia in patients under 55 (British Society of Gastroenterology 2002).

Uncertainty

Family doctors continually have to live with uncertainty and stress in their job as the disease evolves and presents at different stages of its natural history. How far any one family doctor can go depends not only on their training, experience and knowledge of the disease, but also on their own character and to a large extent on the patient's own anxiety and feeling about the illness.

The process of history taking, examination and investigation is all about lessening uncertainty enough to allow a diagnosis to be made and treatment to ensue. As part of that process, it is also important to ask if a particular investigation is likely to alter the management of the problem. A recent article in the *British Medical Journal*, "How many conditions can a family doctor screen for?" (Del and Glasziou 2003) explores the burden of yet another duty that will attract censure if not done properly. Any screening programme to be introduced at community level must fulfil all the criteria set out by Wilson and Junger (1968). Many programmes such as screening for domestic violence would not make any difference to the outcome (Ramsay et al. 2002).

The advantage of primary care is that the care is provided in the community where the patients live and/or work. This enables the patients to report back to the family doctors if the condition changes. Therefore family doctors need to advise patients on how to observe and monitor their condition carefully and when they should report back. For example, a young adult presents to you a vague generalised lower abdominal pain and flu-like illness. On examination there is no localised tenderness or any guarding, and the general condition is good. Your working diagnosis could be viral infection. However you should warn of the possibility of early appendicitis, so the patient needs to observe their condition and report back any worsening of symptoms. By the same token, if the same patient comes in repeatedly, an alarm bell should be ringing for something more serious such as malaria.

In keeping with the hypothetico-deductive method, the "Great Mimickers" can be subdivided into the "Most Likely" and the "Important not to be missed" categories as follows:

Most Likely	Important not to be missed
Anaemia	Chronic Renal Failure
Cancer	Neurological disorders with unusual
Chronic infections: e.g.	presentations: e.g.
TB	Multiple Sclerosis
HIV	Parkinson's Disease
Hepatitis B, C	Guillan-Barre syndrome
Coronary Disease	Atypical Migraine
Depression	SLE and other connective tissue
Diabetes Mellitus	disorders
Drugs:	
Iatrogenic	
Alcohol abuse	
Illicit drug abuse	
Ectopic Pregnancy	
Spinal Dysfunction: pain anywhere in	
the body can emanate from the spine	
Thyroid and other endocrine disorders	
UTI	

(Adopted from John Murtagh *General Practice*. Sydney: McGraw-Hill, 1998.)

Summary

To make a diagnosis in primary care setting, one can:

- Use the hypothetico-deductive method to create a list of:
    - ❖ Most likely diagnoses

❖ Important diagnoses not to be missed

❖ Novelty or rare causes

- Examine the patient to help confirm or refute the most likely diagnoses and important diagnoses

- Put the two together to create the diagnosis or a working diagnosis

- Arrange for appropriate investigations

- Review the situation in the light of time, investigation results and treatment to see if the (working) diagnosis needs to be reviewed or altered

- Always be aware of the limitations of one's own knowledge, capability and expertise and never be afraid to ask colleagues for their opinion because, at the end of the day, it is someone else's life and well-being at stake and the worst that can happen to us is we feel foolish if we make an error

References

British Society of Gastroenterology. 2002. "Dyspepsai management guideline". Retrieved 16 January 2006, from http://www.bsg.org.uk/clinical_prac/guidelines/dyspepsia.htm.

Buchholz, W. J. 1998. "Nonverbal delivery: Some tips on dos and don'ts in public speaking". Retrieved 16 January 2006, from http://web.bentley.edu/empl/b/wbuchholz/presentations/ nonverbal/outlinec.htm.

Cockburn, J. and Pit, S. 1997. "Prescribing behaviour in clinical practice: Patients' expectations and doctors' perceptions of patients' expectations—A questionnaire study". *British Medical Journal*, 315: 520–523.

Comino, E. J., Silove, D., Manicavasagar, V., Harris, E. and Harris, M. F. 2001. "Agreement in symptoms of anxiety and depression between patients and GPs: The influence of ethnicity". *Family Practice*, 18: 71–77.

Del, M. and Glasziou, P. 2003. "How many conditions can a GP screen for?". *British Medical Journal*, 327: 1117.

Greenhalgh, T., Helman, C. and Chowdhury, A. M. 1998. "Health beliefs and folk models of diabetes in British Bangladeshis: A qualitative study". *British Medical Journal*, 316: 978–983.

Griffiths, C., Kaur, G., Gantley, M., Feder, G., Hillier, S., Goddard, J. and

Packe, G. 2001. "Influences on hospital admission for asthma in south Asian and white adults: Qualitative interview study". *British Medical Journal*, 323: 962–966.

Hampton, J. R., Harrison, M. J. B. and Mitchell, J. R. A. 1975. "Relative contributions of history taking, physical examination and laboratory investigation to diagnosis and management of medical outpatients". *British Medical Journal*, 2: 486–489.

Horrocks, S., Anderson, E. and Salisbury, C. 2002. "Systematic review of whether nurse practitioners working in primary care can provide equivalent care to doctors". *British Medical Journal*, 324: 819–823.

Masterson, J. 1996. *Nonverbal Communication in Text-Based Virtual Realities*, Chapter 5. University of Montana. Retrieved January 16, 2006, from http://www.johnmasterson.com/thesis/.

McWhinney, I. 1989. *A Textbook of Family Medicine*. Oxford: Oxford University Press.

Phelan, M., Stradins, L. and Morrison, S. 2001. "Physical health of people with severe mental illness: Can be improved if primary care and mental health professionals pay attention to it". *British Medical Journal*, 322: 443–444.

Ramsay, J., Richardson, J., Carter, Y. H., Davidson, L. L. and Feder, G. 2002. "Should health professionals screen women for domestic violence? Systematic review". *British Medical Journal*, 325: 314–318.

Richards, D., Meakins, J., Tawfik, J., Godfrey, L., Dutton, E., Richardson, G. and Russell, D. 2002. "Nurse telephone triage for same day appointments in general practice: Multiple interrupted time series trial of effect on workload and costs". *British Medical Journal*, 325: 1214.

Sandler, G. 1979. "Costs of unnecessary tests". *British Medical Journal*, 2: 21–24.

Tomlinson, B. and Cockram, C. 2003. "SARS: Experience at Prince of Wales Hospital, Hong Kong". *Lancet*, 361: 1486–1487.

Williams, B., Poulter, N. R., Brown, M. J., Davis, M., McInnes, G. T., Potter, J. F., Sever, P. S. and Thom, S. McG. 2004. "British Hypertension Society guidelines for management of hypertension: Report of the fourth working party of the British Hypertension Society, 2004-BHS IV". *Journal of Human Hypertension*, 18: 139–185.

Wilson, J. M. G. and Junger, J. J. 1968. "Principles and practice of screening for disease". Geneva: World Health Organisation, p. 34.

Chapter 3

Role of Evidence in Primary Care

✑

◆ K. K. TSANG ◆

Scenario

You are a junior medical doctor working in a general outpatient clinic. A 24-year-old man who was discharged from hospital last week following a severe asthma attack came to your office. He had asthma as a child, but prior to this admission he had not experienced any symptoms at all since the age of 14. His medication now includes a salbutamol inhaler for acute shortness of breath and beclometasone (an inhaled steroid). He is a physical fitness trainer and questions you about concerns over his fitness to carry on his job.

Faced with this situation as a trainee family doctor, you were told by your hospital consultant in the past that the risk of dying of asthma at the job was low (although he could not put an exact level on it) and that was the information that should be conveyed to the patient. You now follow this advice, emphasising to the patient the need to continue his medication and to see you in follow up. The patient leaves in a state of vague trepidation about his risk of subsequent asthma attack.

Based on this, is there a need to change our current practices? It has been said that taking an evidence-based approach to practice, teaching and research can help doctors address some of the limitations of current medical practice.

What is evidence-based medicine (EBM)?

One of the most common definitions of EBM comes from Dr. David Sackett who defines EBM as "the conscientious, explicit and judicious use of current best evidence in making decisions about the care of the individual patient. It means integrating individual clinical expertise with the best available external clinical evidence from systematic research." (Sackett 1996).

EBM is the integration of clinical expertise, patient values and the best evidence into the decision-making process for patient care. Clinical expertise refers to the clinician's accumulated experience, education and clinical skills. The patient brings to the encounter their own personal and unique concerns, expectations and values. The best evidence is usually found in clinically relevant research that has been conducted using sound methodology (Sackett et al. 2000). The evidence by itself does not make a decision for you, but it can help support the patient care process. The full integration of these three components into clinical decisions hopes to enhance the opportunity for optimal clinical outcomes and quality of life.

Why is EBM important?

There is good evidence that the quality of care could be better. Such evidence comes from:

- Clinical examples, in which lack of good evidence has led to harm for our patients (Echt et al. 1991)
- Common patterns of thinking introduce bias (Sox et al. 1988)
- There is a wide variation in current clinical practice among physicians (Lu-Yao et al. 1993)
- The difficulty of managing medical information, when results conflict and thousands of articles are published every week
- Our knowledge declines over time, as we get further from medical school, and unfortunately traditional continuous medical education does not work (Sackett et al. 1997)

Evidence-based medicine requires new skills from the clinician, including efficient literature-searching and the application of formal rules of evidence in evaluating clinical literature.

Table 3.1 The steps in the EBM process

The patient	1. Start with the patient—a clinical problem or question arises out of the care of the patient
The question	2. Construct a well-built clinical question derived from the case
The resource	3. Select the appropriate resource(s) and conduct a search
The evaluation	4. Appraise that evidence for its validity (closeness to the truth) and applicability (usefulness in clinical practice)
The patient	5. Return to the patient—integrate that evidence with clinical expertise and patient preferences, and apply it to practice
Self-evaluation	6. Evaluate your performance with this patient

EBM always begins and ends with the patient. To begin this process, consider the previous clinical scenario:

"John is a 24-year-old man discharged from hospital last week following a severe asthma attack. He had asthma as a child, but prior to this admission had not experienced any symptoms at all since the age of 14. His medication now includes a salbutamol inhaler for acute shortness of breath and beclometasone. John is a physical fitness trainer and questions you at his follow-up outpatient appointment about concerns over his fitness to carry on his job."

Anatomy of a good clinical question

Patient or problem

How would you describe a group of patients similar to yours? What are the most important characteristics of the patient? This may include the primary problem, disease or co-existing conditions. Sometimes the sex, age or race of a patient might be relevant to the diagnosis or treatment of a disease if you are sufficiently convinced that the disease will behave differently in these groups.

Intervention, prognostic factor or exposure

Which major interventions, prognostic factors or exposures are you considering? What do you want to do for this patient? To prescribe a drug? To order a test? To refer to your surgical colleagues? What factors may influence the prognosis of the patient? Age? Co-existing problems? What might have precipitated this episode of asthma attack? Asbestos? Cigarette smoke?

Comparison

What are the alternatives when compared to the intervention? For example, are you trying to decide between two drugs or a drug and a placebo, or no medication, or two diagnostic tests? However your clinical question does not always need a specific comparison.

Outcomes

What can you hope to accomplish, measure, improve or affect? What are you trying to do for the patient? To relieve or eliminate the symptoms or the disease? To reduce the number of adverse events? Or to improve function or test scores?

Therefore the structure of the question may look like this:

Patient/Problem	24-year-old male with recurrent asthma
Intervention	Short-acting β-agonist and corticosteroid
Comparison, if any	Other treatments
Outcome	Optimal symptomatic control; prevention of relapse

For our patient, the clinical question could be:

Does the use of a combined salbutamol and beclometasone inhaler for an otherwise young, fit athletic adult provide an optimal symptom control when compared with other treatment regimes?

Two additional elements of the well-built clinical question are the "type of question" (Table 3.2) and the "type of study" (Figure 3.1). This information can be helpful in focusing the question and determining the most appropriate type of evidence.

Table 3.2 The most common types of questions related to clinical tasks

Diagnosis	How to select and interpret diagnostic tests
Therapy	How to select treatments to offer patients that do more good than harm and that are worth the efforts and costs of using them
Prognosis	How to estimate the patient's likely clinical course over time and anticipate likely complications of the disease
Aetiology/Harm	How to identify causes for the disease (including iatrogenic forms)

Figure 3.1 The evidence pyramid showing hierarchy of types of studies

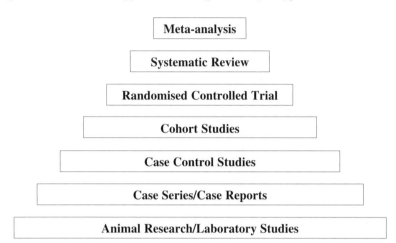

The level of evidence is often referred to as the "evidence pyramid". It is used to illustrate the evolution of the literature. The base of the pyramid is where information usually starts with an idea or laboratory research. As these ideas turn into drugs and diagnostic tools they are tested in laboratory models, then in animals, and finally in humans. The human testing may begin with volunteers and go through several phases of clinical trials before the drug or diagnostic tool can be authorised for use within the general population. Randomised controlled trials (RCT) are then done to further test the effectiveness and efficacy of a drug or therapy. As you move up the pyramid the amount of available literature decreases, but increases in its relevance to the clinical setting.

The type of question is important and can help lead you to the best study design:

Type of Question	Suggested Best Type of Study
Therapy	RCT > cohort > case control > case series
Diagnosis	prospective, blind comparison to a gold standard
Aetiology/Harm	RCT > cohort > case control > case series
Prognosis	cohort > case control > case series
Prevention	RCT > cohort > case control > case series
Clinical Exam	prospective, blind comparison to gold standard
Cost	economic analysis

Our original question, "Does the use of a combined salbutamol and beclometasone inhaler for an otherwise young, fit athletic adult provide an optimal symptom control when compared with other treatment regimes?" is one of therapy, and the best evidence would be a randomised controlled trial. If we find numerous RCTs then we may want to look for a systematic review.

The literature search

Using this question, we will move on to the literature search. Constructing a well-built clinical question can lead directly to a well-built search strategy. Note that you may not use all the pieces of the well-built clinical question in your MEDLINE strategy. For example, we do not include the word therapy. Instead we use the publication type, RCT, to get at the concept of treatment.

The practice of evidence-based medicine advocates that clinicians search the published literature to find answers to their clinical questions. There are literally millions of published reports, journal articles, correspondence and studies available to clinicians. Choosing the best resource to search is an important decision. Large databases such as MEDLINE will give you access to the primary literature. Secondary resources such as ACP Journal Club, POEMS and Clinical Evidence will provide you with an assessment of the original study. The Cochrane Library provides access to systematic reviews which help to summarise the results from a number of studies.

Evaluating the evidence

We have now identified current information which can answer our clinical question. The next step is to read the article and evaluate the study.

There are three basic questions that need to be answered for every type of study:

- Are the results of the study valid?
- What are the results?
- Will the results help in caring for my patient?

The validity criteria should be applied before an extensive analysis of the study data. If the study is not valid, the data may not be useful.

The evidence that supports the validity or truthfulness of the information is found primarily in the study methodology. Here is where the investigators address the issue of bias, both conscious and unconscious.

Evaluating medical literature is a complex undertaking. You may find that the answers to the question of validity may not always be clearly stated in the article and that clinicians will have to make their own judgements about the importance of each question.

Once you have determined that the study methodology is valid, you must examine the results and their applicability to the patient. Clinicians may have additional concerns such as whether the study represented patients similar to theirs, whether the study covered the aspect of the problem that is most important to the patient, or whether the study suggested a clear and useful plan of action.

Return to the patient

To complete the analysis you would need to review the results and determine if they are applicable to your patient, John.

Evaluate your performance

After that, take a moment to reflect on how well you were able to conduct the steps in the EBM process. Did you ask a relevant, well-focused question? Do you have fast and reliable access to the necessary resources? Do you know how to use them efficiently? Did you find a pre-appraised article? If not, was it difficult to critically evaluate the article?

Summary

Based on the limitations of traditional medical practice, a new paradigm for clinical decision-making has arisen. Evidence-based medicine deals with the uncertainties of clinical medicine (an exploding volume of literature, rapid introduction of new technologies, deepening concern about burgeoning medical costs and increasing attention to the quality and outcomes of medical care) and has the potential for transforming the medical education and practice. However evidence-based medicine requires new skills for the physician. Incorporating these skills into both undergraduate and postgraduate medical education will result in more rapid dissemination and integration of the new paradigm into our future medical practice.

References

Echt, D. S., Liebson, P. R., Mitchell, L. B., Peters, R. W., Obias-Manno, D., Barker, A. H., Arensberg, D., Baker, A., Friedman, L., Greene, H. L. et al. 1991. "Mortality and morbidity in patients receiving encainide, flecainide, or placebo. The Cardiac Arrhythmia Suppression Trial". *New England Journal Medicine,* 324: 781–788.

Lu-Yao, G. L., McLerran, D., Wasson, J. and Wennberg, J. E. for the Prostate Patient Ourcomes Research Team. 1993. "An assessment of radical prostatectomy: Time trends, geographic variation, and outcomes". *Journal of American Medical Association,* 269: 2633–2636.

Sackett, D. L. 1996. "Evidence-based medicine—What it is and what it isn't". Retrieved 16 January, 2006, from http://www.cebm.net/ebm_is_isnt.asp.

Sackett, D. L., Richardson, W. S., Rosenberg, W. and Haynes, R. B. (eds.). 1997. *Evidence-based Medicine: How to Practice and Teach EBM* (1st edition). New York: Churchill Livingstone.

Sackett, D. L., Straus, S. E., Richardson, W. S., Rosenberg, W. and Haynes, R. B. 2000. *Evidence-based Medicine: How to Practice and Teach EBM* (2nd edition). Edinburgh: Churchill Livingstone.

Sox, H. C., Blatt, M. A., Higgins, M. C. and Marton, K. I. 1988. *Medical Decision Making* (2nd edition). New York: Butterworths.

Chapter 4

Management of Chronic Illnesses

◆ Kenny KUNG, Augustine LAM, Philip K. T. LI ◆

Background

Our population is ageing. It is anticipated that by mid-2021 the number of senior citizens will reach 1.4 million, accounting for 17.2% of the Hong Kong population (Census and Statistics Department 2002; Department of Health 2004). Chronic diseases are expected to become the major cause of morbidity and mortality, as well as an increasing burden for healthcare resources (Murray and Lopez 1996). Particular diseases identified by the World Health Organization (WHO) include diabetes mellitus, hypertension, asthma, chronic obstructive airway disease, coronary heart disease, dyslipidaemia, mental health disorders such as depression, and certain communicable diseases such as HIV infection (Epping-Jordan et al. 2001). In Hong Kong, patients with diabetes accounted for more than 15,000 hospital admissions, cerebrovascular disease (25,000) and heart disease (60,000) (Centre for Health Protection 2005) in 2000.

Definition

It is difficult to define what chronic illness is. The term "chronic" stems from the Greek word "chronos", meaning time. Therefore it is obvious that chronic illnesses are those that persist with time. Although stakeholders in the healthcare system have been unable to reach a consensus as to its definition (Carter et al. 2002), various concepts associated with "chronic illness" have been proposed. Invariably, they possess the following characteristics:

- Are ongoing and problematic to patients, and may lead to disability
- May fluctuate, be episodic and progressive
- Are incurable but may be controllable
- Affect quality of life and involve making lifestyle changes, such as changing job duties
- Impact on relationships, e.g. family and employment
- Contain elements of uncertainty, e.g. of future needs, recurrence
- Are expensive to treat
- Require ongoing and complex management, including medical, personal care, community support, self-management programmes and multi-disciplinary approaches
- May be serious and complicated, and produce multiple problems in terms of medical care and management.

Perhaps though, the biggest negative effect is that on doctors. When talking about chronic illness the feelings of hopelessness, "nothing can be done" and professional impotence are conjured up. The reality is that the biggest test of a caring profession and the most interesting challenges come from treating these patients (note: we did not use the term illness; for it is by de-personalising the patient that much of the criticism of the medical profession stems). It is only in American TV programmes where doctors are rushing around that medicine seems so acute and exciting. Once you have dealt with an asthma or heart attack a few times you will find that they are not particularly difficult to handle. On the other hand *preventing* the asthma attack can be far harder and as a consequence more rewarding both professionally and for the patients too. A sincere thank you from a patient or their relative makes us all beam.

It is this attitudinal change and the realisation that the vast bulk of our work is to do with chronic illnesses that have lead many in the UK to now use the term "Long-Term Condition". In itself it will not lead to better patient care but if it does lead to an altered and more positive view from the medical profession then it would have succeeded. Similarly talking about patients with, say, diabetes rather than a diabetic patient may seem pedantic, trivial or political correctness gone mad but again it is about changing attitudes to the positive.

Principles of management

Management of chronic illnesses is tough but often more rewarding than other aspects of medicine. Poor patient prognosis, working under pressure, feeling overwhelmed by the chronicity of the illness and the complexity of symptoms, the lack of time and the problems of patient compliance makes the management of chronic illnesses difficult (Proudfoot et al. 2002). In order to provide effective management, it is necessary to have good basic knowledge of the principles of family medicine and then apply these to the management plan of chronic illnesses. Brian McAvoy's helpful mnemonic "RAPRIOP" (Fraser and McAvoy 1992) is quite useful as a simple aid. It stands for:

Reassurance

Advice

Prescription

Referral

Investigation

Observation (follow up)

Prevention

Every management decision should also be guided by two other basic principles of family medicine, namely the tripartite model of disease comprising biological, psychological and social aspects of the problem, as well as consideration of the short-term, intermediate-term and long-term management.

Biopsychosocial model of chronic illness and progression with time

To be diagnosed with a chronic illness is just the beginning of a long journey for the patient. It is a label allowing oneself to be grouped so that treatment can be standardised, and allowing authorities to collect epidemiological data. But what does it mean to the individual?

Since health involves a state of physical, psychological and social well-being, chronic illness can also be viewed as a dysfunction of any or a combination of these three components. There is an ongoing interaction between a chronic disease and an individual. The importance of these interactions may vary with time. A disease may not result in any symptoms initially, but as it progresses, symptoms and complications as a result of the disease as well as treatment will follow. Therefore particular emphasis must be given to predict disease progress and to arrange management plans at the short-, intermediate- and long-term levels. Table 4.1 illustrates examples of management plans for three common chronic diseases.

Although it seems artificial to categorise management in a time-limiting fashion, this method helps the family doctor to appreciate chronic disease as a function of time. As mentioned previously, chronic illness is by definition ongoing and may continue to be a problem for the patient and the family. As a patient gets older, their status in the family life cycle and societal role will change. Our body's biological and psychological status is closely linked with our social functioning, as depicted by the overlapping circles in Figure 4.1. Indeed, a change in any of the three basic functions of the biopsychosocial model will cause a change in the other functions. Because of this closely-linked relationship, a plan that involves short- to long-term goals will provide holistic bases for the care of the patient.

Emphasis on the biopsychosocial model is important. Modern medicine has become too system-based, further perpetuated by the widespread use of disease classification systems, and this is something we are trying to avoid in this textbook. Effective management can only occur if we perceive illness from the patients' perspective, understanding how the illness has affected them physically and how they relate these

Figure 4.1 Interface of physical, psychological and social function in chronic illness

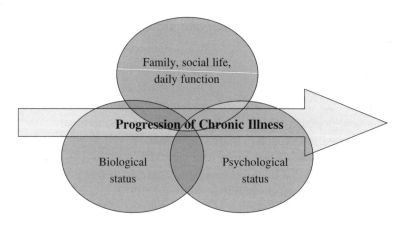

Table 4.1 Management of common chronic disorders using short-/intermediate-/long-term management plans and RAPRIOP model

Disease	Management Plan		
	Short-term	Intermediate-term	Long-term
Diabetes Mellitus	Disease education Lifestyle promotion Screen for: – complications – other associated illnesses	Home monitoring techniques Consider drug therapy Assessing home and family situation Drug compliance	Screen for: – complications – other associated illnesses Drug compliance Impact on work and other social issues
	Reassurance – if good control, risk of complications reduced Advice – education on foot care, diet, exercise, travel particularly if using insulin, hypoglycemia Prescription – when diet control inadequate Referral – when control with drugs inadequate, or if presence of complications	Investigation – annual check (fundi, HbA1c, ECG, urine) Observation (follow up) – regular follow up Prevention – prevent onset of cardiovascular diseases through lifestyle modification and/or medications, flu vaccinations, medication side-effects, impotence, triopathy	
Coronary heart disease	Disease education Lifestyle promotion Initiate drug treatment Screen for: – complications – other associated illnesses	Education on nitrate use Education for relatives Consider specialist referral Drug compliance	Screen for: – complications – other associated illnesses Impact on work and other social issues Drug compliance
	Reassurance Advice – quit smoking, diet, exercise, travel advice Prescription – regular + as needed, education on use Referral – to specialist when inadequate control	Investigation – to consider invasive management Observation (follow up) – regular follow up Prevention – quit smoking, flu vaccinations, medication side-effects	
Chronic obstructive airway disease	Symptom-relief with bronchodilators Inhaler education Disease education Lifestyle promotion Smoking advice	Pulmonary rehabilitation Education on exacerbations Drug compliance Inhaler technique	Screen for: – complications – other associated illnesses Impact on work and other social issues Drug compliance Consider need for long-term and/or ambulatory oxygen therapy
	Reassurance Advice – quit smoking, exercise, breathing techniques Prescription – ensure puffer technique, use of accessories Referral – to physiotherapy, occupation therapy, specialist when inadequate control	Investigation – important during exacerbations Observation (follow up) – regular follow up, may increase frequency in winter Prevention – quit smoking, flu vaccinations, plasma drug levels (theophyllines)	

discomforts to the illness. Showing genuine empathy simply cannot be over-emphasised. Patients must be made aware that we understand how they feel. No matter how difficult their individual situations may be, we need to reassure them that they are not alone in fighting their chronic illness. As their family doctors, we must provide them with adequate explanation and education so that they realise that their individual experience is shared by many others having the same illness. Patient support groups and written materials are tremendously helpful for patients to understand this concept.

Patients entering our consultation room with any illness have literally surrendered their private information to our care. They have willingly given up control over their health when seeking for our advice. Therefore whenever possible it is always useful to return this disease management "control" to the patients, i.e. getting the patient to take back ownership. Examples of this include home blood glucose monitoring, home blood pressure monitoring and home peak flow rate measurement. Although studies have shown that some of these interventions may not improve clinical outcome, they certainly do increase patients' knowledge and enhance their self-awareness about their disease.

Pharmacological intervention is often the major component in chronic illness management. Most medications aim to improve biological and psychological well-being. However all medications have side-effects, including placebo. It is our duty to provide patients with the necessary information with regard to possible side-effects, but without scaring them off from taking these drugs. In a significant proportion of patients, poor drug compliance is a recurrent problem. However by getting patients to take ownership of their illness in part by discussing with them various management options including the use of drugs when indicated, compliance, can be improved. If I tell you to do something would you do it? May be, may be not. If you agree to do it, you will (assuming your word is your bond). Adequate explanation, keeping the regimen simple and helping patients adapt to drug intake with daily routines are also essential to improve compliance.

Wider perspective of chronic illness

Although the impact of chronic illness is significant to individual patients, solely addressing issues from the patients' perspective will only solve part of the problem. Family doctors act as the gatekeepers for our healthcare system and are the major coordinators of healthcare resources. Indeed family doctors have been identified as being able to deal with uncertainty and with patients having complex and multiple problems (Royal College of General Practitioners 2004). Countries where primary care is driven by family doctors have reported better health outcomes and cost performance (Macinko et al. 2003). Having ready access to effective primary care also offers the potential to reduce disparities in care, increasing opportunities to live healthily and productively (Schoen et al. 2004). Family doctors are, therefore, not only essential to individual patient's care but also to any healthcare infrastructure.

From the above discussion, it is clear that chronic illnesses should be tackled not only at an individual level but also at a population level. Population-based management does not target a specific patient, but aims to reduce the impact of chronic illnesses in the community through disease prevention and risk reduction. The philosophy is that if the population is healthier, then there will be less illness around, and hence a lesser burden on our society.

Disease prevention from the family doctor's perspective is much more than the traditional skills of management (diagnosis, treatment and the prescribing of medications) learnt in medical school. As family doctors see their patients on average three to four times a year, they are often in the best position to practise their skills in prevention, including vaccination, contraception, risk assessment, counselling, lifestyle modification through health education (primary prevention), identification of disease at the presymptomatic stage (secondary prevention), as well as complication reduction (tertiary prevention).

In order to ensure the best utilisation of our limited resources, population-based strategies must involve prioritisation. However to decide how to allocate resources to one individual but deny them to another is a subject of controversy. Health authorities continually need to balance the need for treatment, the benefit treatment can bring, value for money and community values in their management decisions (Shaw 1996; Bill 1996). Family doctors are not exempt from this balancing act. Indeed, since we work for the best interests of the majority of our population, efficient rationalisation has to be introduced.

Certain chronic illnesses have guidelines to ensure rational management. These conditions are usually those that are prevalent in our society and whose treatment incurs high costs. The management of dyslipidaemia is an example. Studies have demonstrated the benefits of targeting lipid levels with statins and fibrates to a certain extent (Pedersen et al. 1996; Jukema et al. 1995). Furthermore drug trials have also highlighted the benefits of primary prevention in patients with dyslipidaemia (Shepherd et al. 1995). Despite the multitude of high quality trial evidence, translation of trial data to the general population has not been implemented in many countries. The British national policy is to only provide statin therapy for those with a coronary heart disease risk of 10– 15% or more (Prodigy guidance). In Hong Kong, the Hospital Authority has taken a similar stand (Hospital Authority 2005).

Finally, ongoing research at a local level forms an integral part of future disease management. Learning from overseas and hospital specialist experience is essential, but ethnic differences and population diversity may render certain evidence non-applicable to the local primary care population. Local research in family medicine therefore provides a platform to capture data from the local primary care population, as well as to review and improve current healthcare provision.

Summary

Providing an effective management plan for patients with chronic illnesses is not an easy task. Historical development in Hong Kong has helped to merge Chinese and Western cultures. Health-seeking behaviour in our population has undergone similar integration. Many patients seek advice from traditional Chinese medicine practitioners whilst they concurrently receive Western types of treatment, and vice versa. Within the public healthcare setting, information continuity has been facilitated by the development of a region-wide computerised clinical management system. Futher integration of patient information through secure public-private interface systems will help to ensure complete continuity while preserving confidentiality.

The public in Hong Kong has unrestricted access to medical information from the media and Internet. However unfiltered medical information may affect the management plan rather than promote compliance. Further to this is the problem of "doctor shopping", that is, patients changing their family doctors when their expectations, reasonably or otherwise, are not met. Patient education for establishing a trusting doctor-patient relationship plays a crucial role in counterbalancing these drawbacks. Although such education is essential in our day-to-day patient encounters, of equal importance is to educate the public, providing them with the necessary and appropriate knowledge. Only through increasing patient empowerment can our resources be effectively and efficiently utilised without causing dissent from patients.

References

Carter, M., Walker, C. and Furler, J. 2002. "Developing a shared meaning of chronic illness: The implications and benefits for general practice". *General Practice Evaluation Program (GPEP) Project Summary.*

Census and Statistics Department. 2002. *Hong Kong Population Projections 2002–2031.*

Department of Health. 2004. *Elderly Health, Topical Health Report No. 3.*

Department of Health, Centre for Health Protection, Hong Kong. 2005. *Non-communicable disease.*

Epping-Jordan, J., Bengoa, R., Kawar, R. and Sabate, E. 2001. "The challenge of chronic conditions: WHO responds". *British Medical Journal*, 323: 947–948.

Fraser, R. C. and McAvoy, B. 1992. *Clinical Method, a General Practice Approach* (2nd edition). Oxford: Butterworth-Heinemann, pp. 59–76.

Hospital Authority. 2005. *HA Drug Formulary 2005.*

Jukema, J. W., Bruschke, A. V. G., Van Boven A. J., Reiber, J. H. C. , Bal. E. T., Zwinderman, A. H., Jansen, H., Boerma, G. J. M., Van Rappard, F. M. and Lie, K. I. 1995 . "Effect of lipid lowering by pravastatin on progression and regression of coronary artery disease in symptomatic men with normal to moderately elevated serum cholesterol levels: The Regression Growth Evaluation Statin Study (REGRESS)". *Circulation*, 91: 2528–2540.

Kung K., Lam, A. and Li, P. K. T. 2004. "Survey on the disease spectrum encountered by family medicine trainees". WONCA 2004, 3482, abstract p. 143.

Kung K., Lam, A. and Li, P. K. T. 2005. "The use and efficacy of statins in Hong Kong Chinese dyslipidaemic patients in a primary care setting". *Hong Kong Practitioner*, 27: 450–454.

Kung K., Lam, A. and Li, P. K. T. "Management of common conditions—A comparative study of family physicians and medical physicians". Health Authority Convention 2007. SPP-P5.41. Abstract p. 44.

Macinko, J, Starfield and B, Shi. L. 2003. "The contribution of primary care systems to health outcomes within Organization for Economic Cooperation and Development (OECD) countries, 1970–1998". *Health Services Research,* 38, no. 3: 831–865.

Murray, C. J. L. and Lopez, A. D. (eds.). 1996. *The Global Burden of Disease: A Comprehensive Assessment of Mortality and Disability from Diseases, Injuries, and Risk Factors in 1990 and Projected to 2020.* Cambridge, MA: Harvard University Press.

New, B. 1996."The rationing agenda in the NHS". *British Medical Journal,* 312: 1593–1601.

Pedersen, T. R, Berg, K, Cook, T. J, Faergeman, O., Haghfelt, T., Kjekshus, J., Miettinen, T., Musliner, T. A., Olsson, A. G., Pyörälä, K., Thorgeirsson, G., Tobert, J. A., Wedel, H. and Wilhelmsen, L. 1996. "Safety and tolerability of cholesterol lowering with simvastatin during 5 years in the Scandinavian simvastatin survival study". *Archives Internal Medicine,* 156: 2085.

Prodigy guidance. United Kingdom.

Proudfoot, J., Infante, J. O., Davies, G. P. and Harris, M. 2002. *The Challenges GPs Face in Providing Good Chronic Disease Management. Living Better: Towards a Better Quality of Life.* Annual Scientific Convention, Perth, Australia, 5–9 October 2002.

Royal College of General Practitioners. 2004. *The Future of General Practice.* London: Royal College of General Practitioners.

Schoen, C., Osborn, R., Huynh, P. T., Doty, M., Davis, K., Zapert, K. and Peugh, J. 2004. "Primary care and health system performance: Adults' experiences in five countries". *Health Systems Primary Care Web Exclusive.*

Shaw, A. B. 1996. "Age as a basis for healthcare rationing: Support for agist policies". *Drugs Aging,* 9 (6): 403–405.

Shepherd, J., Cobbe, S, M., Ford, I., Isles, C. G., Lorimer, A. R., Macfarlane, P. W., McKillop, J. H. and Packard, C. J. 1995. "Prevention of coronary heart disease with pravastatin in men with hypercholesterolemia". *New England Journal of Medicine,* 333: 1301–1307.

Chapter 5

Effective Lifestyle Changes

✑

◆ Albert LEE ◆

Importance of lifestyle changes

Chronic illnesses are now the major cause of death and disability worldwide. Non-communicable diseases (NCD) such as cardiovascular disease (CVD), diabetes, obesity, cancer and respiratory diseases account for 59% of the 56.5 million deaths annually and 45.9% of the global burden of disease (WHO 2002). A second wave of epidemic of cardiovascular disease is hitting developing countries hard due to a change of lifestyles (Murray and Lopez 1996). Death and disability from ischaemic heart diseases and cerebrovascular accidents rank number one and four respectively. Cancer accounts for a further 7.1 million deaths annually (12.6% of the global total). Dietary factors account for 30% of all cancers in Western countries, and approximately up to 20% in developing countries (second to tobacco as preventable cause). The number of new cases of cancer is estimated to increase from 10 million annually to 15 million by 2020.

A few risk factors are responsible for the majority of these chronic illnesses. In a recent article in *Lancet*, the researchers concluded, "abnormal lipids, smoking, hypertension, diabetes, abdominal obesity, psychosocial factors, consumption of fruits, vegetables and alcohol, and regular physical activity account for most of the risk of myocardial infarction worldwide in both sexes and at all ages in all regions." (Yusulf et al. 2004). Nine risk factors have been identified as accounting for 90% of the population attributable risk (PAR) in men and 94% in women (Yusulf et al. 2004) and they are:

- Smoking (odds ratio [OR] 2.87 for current vs. never, PAR 35.7% for current and former vs. never)
- Raised ApoB/ApoA1 ratio (OR 3.25 for top vs. lowest quintile, PAR 49.2% for top four quintiles vs. lowest quintile)
- History of hypertension (OR 1.91, PAR 17.9%)
- Diabetes (OR 2.37, PAR 9.9%)
- Abdominal obesity (OR 1.12 for top vs. lowest tertile and 1.62 for middle vs. lowest tertile, PAR 20.1% for top two tertiles vs. lowest tertile)
- Psychosocial factors (OR 2.67, PAR 32.5%)
- Daily consumption of fruits and vegetables (OR 0.70, PAR 13.7% for lack of daily consumption)
- Regular alcohol consumption (OR 0.91, PAR 6.7%)
- Regular physical activity (OR 0.86, PAR 12.2%)

All the above were significantly related to acute myocardial infarction ($p < 0.0001$ for all risk factors and $p = 0.03$ for alcohol).

These associations were noted in men and women, old and young, and in all regions of the world. Putting it another way: compared to non-smokers, 58% of lung cancer deaths, 37% of chronic obstructive pulmonary disease deaths, 20% of tuberculosis deaths and 23% of vascular deaths could have been avoided (Sitas et al. 2004).

Another study found that high intake of red and processed meat was associated with higher risk of colon cancer (after adjusting for age and energy intake) but not after further adjustments for body mass index, cigarette smoking and other covariates (Chao et al. 2005). When long-term consumption was considered, persons in the highest percentile of consumption of processed meat had a higher risk of distal colon cancer (OR 1.50) whilst high consumption of red meat was associated with higher risk of rectal cancer (OR 1.71; $p = 0.007$ for trend). Conversely, long-term consumption of poultry and fish was inversely associated with risks of both proximal and distal colon cancer. The researchers concluded that prolonged high consumption of red and processed meat might increase the risk of cancer in the distal portion of the large intestine.

Obesity is linked to many health conditions in older people such as diabetes mellitus (DM), knee replacements, hypertension, pancreatitis, chronic fatigue and insomnia (Patterson et al. 2004). There is a great deal of evidence that both genetic and environmental factors are of importance in the pathogenesis of type 2 diabetes (Uusitupa 2002). Physical inactivity, high fat diet and diet rich in saturated fats all increase risks of DM (WHO 1994; Hu et al. 2001; Vessby et al. 2001) and thus an increase in physical activity and moderate weight loss will help to reduce the incidence of type 2 diabetes by 50% in middle-aged men with impaired glucose tolerance (IGT) (Eriksson and Lindgarde 1991). In a Chinese study of glucose intolerant patients, a 6-year intervention with diet and physical activity resulted in 30–40% reduction in diabetes risks in both normal and overweight persons.

Fifty per cent of premature deaths are related to risk behaviours and 70% of disease burdens and costs are due to these risk behaviours. Therefore a change in dietary habits, physical activity and tobacco control will have a major impact in reducing the rates of these chronic illnesses, surprisingly in a relatively short time. There is overwhelming evidence that prevention is possible when sustained actions are directed both at individuals and families; as well as the broader social, economic and cultural determinants of NCD. However to get a person to change their life-long habits is no easy task and requires strong self-motivation as well as support, both from the family and health professionals.

Behavioural counselling, which is based on social learning theory and the stages of change model, is regarded as an appropriate method of encouraging change in behaviour. Interventions are tailored to an individual with personalised specific advice and setting of short- and long-term goals, depending on the motivational readiness of the individual. Effective lifestyle changes cannot be achieved by just instilling expert knowledge alone. Family doctors need to be equipped with the skills to motivate patients to adopt a healthy lifestyle. This chapter will discuss various strategies for promoting healthy lifestyles to our patients in the family medicine setting.

Models and theories behind behavioural change

People's behaviour is partly determined by their attitudes to that behaviour. An individual's attitude to a specific action and the intention for modification are influenced by beliefs, a motivation which derives from the person's values, experience and instincts as well as the influences from social norms. In Social Learning Theory it is suggested that the ways in which people explain the things happening to them is a product of their childhood experiences. Those who are rewarded for their successes and punished consistently and fairly will come to believe that they are in control of their lives. Those who have inconsistent rewards or punishments irrespective of their behaviour are more likely to see events as a consequence of chance and their own role as irrelevant (Rotter 1954).

Control can be understood in terms of:

- Internal locus of control (the extent to which individuals believe that they are responsible for their own health)
- External locus of control (people who believe that their actions are influenced by powerful others, chance, fate or such)

Those having a strong internal locus of control will see themselves as more able to act decisively and capably. People with external locus of control would be those with lower levels of education so they might not perceive themselves as having much control over their lives or health status. Conversely, people with internal locus of control are usually more educated so they would undertake more preventive health actions or change to more healthy behaviour.

As we can see, the simple model of Knowledge-Attitudes-Behaviour cannot explain behavioural change. Information alone is neither necessary nor sufficient for changing people's behaviour. Most people are aware of the health risks of smoking, but still a substantial proportion of the population continues to smoke.

Values that are acquired through recognition and emotionally adapted beliefs make up what a person thinks of as being important. A whole range of feelings about family, friendships, career and life expectation will influence one's values. Attitudes are more specific than values in describing relatively stable feelings towards a particular issue. Changing attitudes may stimulate behavioural change but, at the same time, behavioural change may influence attitudes. For example, people will still drink alcohol despite a negative attitude towards drinking, but once they have stopped they may develop negative views on drinking.

Attitudes are made up of two components:

- Cognitive: The knowledge and information they possess
- Affective: The feelings, emotions and the evaluation of importance

Attitudes are not easy to change. "Cognitive dissonance" describes a person's mental state when the new information is contradictory to what is already held (Festinger 1957). People either reject the new information as unreliable or inappropriate, or adopt behavioural change that fits with it. Therefore people *can* change their behaviour with new information alone. When an action becomes enjoyable, people will be more motivated and a behavioural change will follow.

Tones (1994) used the term "drive" in the Health Action Model to describe strong motivating factors such as hunger, thirst, sex and pain. It can also be used to describe motivations which can become drives such as addiction. The role of modelling has been particularly important in health promotion, e.g. indirect modelling of the behaviour through the media. Models with status and credibility such as musicians, sportsmen and opinion leaders can be used to present health promotion messages. Social Learning Theory uses the term "instinct" to describe behaviours, which are not learnt but are present at birth (Bandura 1977). Instincts can override attitudes and beliefs. For example, hunger can easily override a person's attitude towards diet. Social Learning Theory further suggests that people make choices in relation to:

- Outcome expectations (whether an action will lead to a particular outcome)
- Self efficacy (whether people believe they can change)

Perception of self-efficacy are based on their assessment as to whether they have the knowledge skills to make changes in their behaviour and also whether external factors such as time and money will allow the change. Many health education programmes, especially those for young people, focus on development of self-concept and self-esteem to equip young people with efficacy skills to resist peer group pressure and increase self-awareness.

The Social Cognition Model, however, highlights the important points on attitudes:

- People's views about the cause and prevention of ill health
- The extent to which people feel that they can control their life and make changes
- Whether they believe change is necessary
- Whether change is perceived to be beneficial in the long run, outweighing any difficulties and problems that may be involved

These models recognise that what people say is not necessary a guide to what they will do and that there are numerous antecedent and situational variables.

The Health Belief Model (Figure 5.1) suggests that whether people change their behaviour or not depends on their evaluation of feasibility and the benefits gained weighed against the costs (Rosenstock 1966; Becker 1974). For people to change their behaviour, they:

- Must have an incentive to change
- Feel threatened by their current behaviour
- Feel a change to be beneficial in some aspect with few adverse consequences
- Feel competent to adopt the change

Individuals are influenced by how vulnerable they perceive themselves to be to an illness or injury, its severity and their susceptibility. The perceptions of risk in older people are very different from in younger ones as risk taking is part of youth development. Therefore it is harder for

Figure 5.1 Health Belief Model (Rosenstock 1966; Becker 1974)

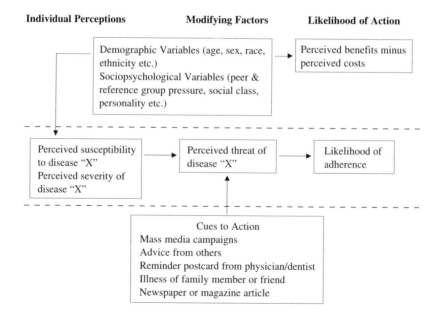

young people to appreciate the long-term effects of smoking, unhealthy eating habits and so on.

Many health education campaigns motivate people to change behaviour through fear or guilt. However the negative attitude resulting from fear disappears over time. It only works if the threat is (and continues to be) perceived as serious and likely to materialise if the advice is not followed.

In the Health Belief Model, people need to have some cues in order to take action for behaviour change and the issue needs to be salient or relevant. This could be changes in one's internal state, e.g. a patient stops smoking with a respiratory infection as smoking makes the cough worse. It could be an external factor, e.g. change in circumstance such as change in job, or death or illness of a close relative or friend. It could also be comments from a significant person such as health care professionals. The family doctor has the advantage of expertise, trust and authority to motivate patients to change behaviour.

The Health Belief Model has been criticised for the lack of weighting in a number of factors—all cues to preventive action. Behavioural change is complex and can be explained by summing up all the different parts via analysis of a set of conceptual components isolated from one another. Ajen and Fishbein's (1980) Theory of Reasoned Action suggested two dependent variables for a behaviour, which forms an intention for change (Figure 5.2):

Figure 5.2 Theory of Reasoned Action (Ajen and Fishbein 1980)

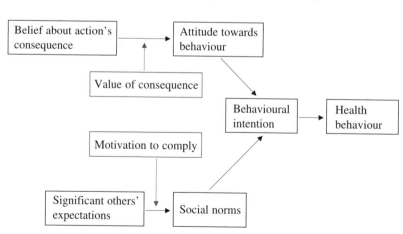

- Attitudes: Beliefs about the consequences of the behaviour and an appraisal of the positive and negative aspects of making a change
- Subjective norms: What "significant others" do and expect, and the degree to which the person wants to conform with others

However people do not always behave consistently with their intentions. The ability to predict behaviour is influenced by the stability of a person's belief, and stability is determined by strength of belief and how long it has been held and is also reinforced by peer groups. The Theory of Reasoned Action places importance on social norms as a major influence on behaviour.

Making a change

Family doctors have taken on the role of assessment and advice in brief interventions (Rollnick et al. 1992). There are guidelines to identify those at risk so family doctors can try to encourage clients to change those aspects of their behaviour (http://www.csu.med.cuhk.edu.hk/~dfm/ p_guideline/). Prochaska and DiClemente (1984, 1986) developed a stage model of behaviour acquisition showing that any change is not final but is an ongoing cycle of change (Figure 5.3). The model helps to reassure healthcare professionals that a relapse on their patients' part is not necessarily a failure and that they can go backwards and forwards. As a family doctor, we can focus on any particular step towards a lifestyle change and provide the patient with a sense of achievement. This model

Figure 5.3 Stages of change model (Prochaska and DiClemente 1984)

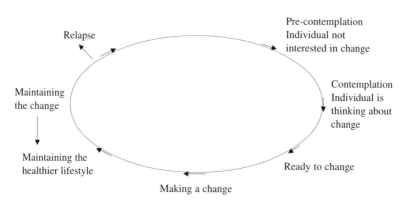

will help the patient to be more involved in the planning process, which in turn makes them more motivated (MacLeod and Dines 1993).

For example, it is important to know if the patient is not yet ready for change (the pre-contemplative stage) and so all the healthcare professional can do is offer support and advise him/her to return if they change their mind. This model explains how people change rather than why they change.

The prerequisites for behaviour change

If a person processes certain qualities or is under certain conditions, their behavioural change is more likely to succeed (RUHBC 1989):

- The change must be self-initiated

- The behaviour must become salient, e.g. a life event such as death of relative from lung cancer might prompt smoking cessation

- The salience of behaviour must appear over a long period of time

- The behaviour is not part of individual's coping strategies, i.e. patients need to develop other coping strategies (patients using smoking for stress management will need to try other relaxation exercise)

- Ideally, there should not be any overwhelming concurrent life issues, e.g. the person concerned has multiple problems such as poverty and concurrent relationship issues

- Availability of social support (WHO [1987] recognised the important role of the health promoter in stimulating and maintaining social support for individuals and groups)

Implementing a plan for change

If a person has some of the above qualities and is ready to take some action (contemplation stage), we can help by, for example, in quitting smoking:

- Goal-setting

- Learn about nicotine addiction and withdrawal, and ways to quit

- Prepare for a quit plan: gradual/abrupt; with or without nicotine replacement or help from outside agency

- Establishing contract: make a mutual contract to support each other in securing measurable and lasting behavioral change

- Inform family and friends

- Acknowledge difficulties (e.g. in face of stress) and high failure rate whilst reinforcing patient's motivational reasons for change

Following through

Once the patient engages in a behavioural change (action/maintenance stage), it is important to continue to motivate them through follow up and support. The doctor may:

- Provide a rationale for follow up (*"I think it is important for you to come and discuss [choose one of the following:] how to overcome nicotine addiction or deal with the complications from your smoking"*)
- Clarify reason for attending follow up (*"Why is it important to attend a follow-up appointment?"* Or *"What health concerns do you want to address at your next appointment?"*)
- Arrange follow up (*"How soon do you want to come back and check up on your concern?"*)

Preventing relapse

Patients who maintain a lifestyle change are found to have similar skills for coping with stress; the difference is that people who relapse failed to use these skills at the time of need. Studies that have examined relapse prevention strategies are, at best, moderately encouraging. In the follow up, some strategies for maintaining quitting smoking are listed below:

- Management of risk situations, e.g. Discuss the previous circumstances when this patient relapsed into smoking and make a list of ways to deal with the urges and cravings
- Pharmacological management, e.g. Explore concerns regarding use of nicotine replacement
- Emotional management, e.g. Stress management
- Re-evaluation of supports
- Re-evaluation of barriers, e.g. Discuss difficulties in quitting smoking and handling techniques
- Use of positive encouragement, e.g. Search for a reward appropriate for the patient

Summary

In summary, different models point out that there are factors accounting for health behaviour change and they are:

- Perception of risk and vulnerability
- Perception of the severity of the disease
- Perceived effectiveness of the behaviour in contributing to better health
- Perception of own ability to make a change
- Perception of how significant others evaluate the behaviour

For behaviour change, a family doctor has the role of providing patients with the knowledge and skills, minimising the barriers to positive health and inequalities of health, and providing an environment that makes healthy choice an easier one.

The *World Health Report 1997* (WHO 1997) indicated priorities for action that are intended to improve mankind's ability to prevent, treat, rehabilitate and, where possible, cure major NCD and to reduce the enormous suffering and disability that they cause. It stated that, as many of the diseases shared a relatively small number of crucial risk factors, an integrated, coordinated approach to their prevention is therefore necessary. There is an urgent need to raise awareness of and motivation for healthy lifestyles.

References

Ajen, I. 1991. "The theory of planned behaviours". *Organisational Behaviour and Human Decision Processes*, 50: 179–211.

Ajen, I. and Fishbein, M. 1980. *Understanding Attitudes and Predicting Behaviours*. Englewood Cliffs: Prentice Hall.

Bandura, A. 1977. *Social Learning Theory*. Englewood Cliffs: Prentice Hall.

Becker, M. H. (ed.). 1974. *The Health Belief Model and Personal Health Behaviour*. New Jersey: Slack, Thorofare.

Chao, A., Michael, J., Thun, M. J., Cari, J., Connell, C. J., Marjorie, L., McCullough, M. L., Jacobs, E. J., Flanders, D., Rodriguez, C., Sinha, R. and Calle, E. E. 2005. "Meat consumption and risk of colorectal cancer". *Journal of American Medical Association*, 293: 172–182.

Eriksson, K. F. and Lindgarde, F. 1991. "Prevention of type 2 (non-insulin dependent) diabetes mellitus by diet and physical exercise: The 6-year Malmo feasibility study". *Diabetologia*, 34: 891–980.

Festinger, L. 1957. *A Theory of Cognitive Dissonance*. Stanford: Stanford University Press.

Hu, F. B., van Dam, R. M. and Liu, S. 2001. "Diet and risk of type 2 diabetes: the role of types of fat and carbohydrate". *Diabetologia*, 44: 805–817.

MacLeod, C. J. and Dines, A. 1993. "Nurses working with people who wish to stop smoking". In Dines, A. and Cribb, A. (eds.) *Health Promotion: Concepts and Practice*. Oxford: Blackwell, pp. 67–84.

Murray, C. J. L. and Loppz, A. D. 1996. *The Global Burden of Disease*. WHO.

Patterson, R. E., Frank, L. L., Kristal, A. R. and White, E. 2004. "A comprehensive examination of health conditions associated with obesity in older adults". *American Journal of Preventive Medicine*, 27 (5): 385–390.

Prochaska, J. O. and DiClemente, C. C. 1984. *The Transtheoretical Approach: Crossing Traditional Foundation of Change*. Homewood, IL: Don Jones/ Irwin.

———. 1986. "Towards a comprehensive model of change". *American Psychologist*, 47: 1102–1114.

Rollnick, S., Heather, N. and Bell, A. 1992. "Negotiating behaviour change in medical settings: The development of brief motivational interviewing". *Journal of Mental Health,* 1: 25–37.

Rosenstock, I. 1966. "Why people use health services". *Millbank Memorial Fund Quarterly*, 44: 94–121.

Rotter, J. B. 1954. *Social Learning and Clinical Psychology*. Englewood Cliffs, NJ: Prentice Hall.

RUHBC (Research Unit in Health and Behaviour Change). 1989. *Changing the Public Health*. Chichester: Wiley, chapter 5.

Sitas, F., Urban, M., Bradshaw, D., Kielkowski, D., Bah, S. and Peto, R. 2004. "Tobacco attributable deaths in South Africa". *Tobacco Control*, 13: 396– 399.

Tones, K. and Tilford, S. 1994. *Health Education: Effectiveness, Efficiency and Equity*. London: Chapman and Hall.

Uusitupa, M. 2002. "Lifestyles matter in the prevention of type 2 diabetes". *Diabetes Care*, 25 (9): 1650–1651.

Vessby, B., Uusitupa, M., Hermansen, K., Riccardi, G., Rivellese, A. A., Tapsell, L. C., Nälsén, G., Berglund, L., Louheranta, A., Rasmussen, B. M., Calvert, G. D., Maffetone, A., Pedersen, E., Gustafsson, I. B. and Storlien, L. H. 2001. "Substituting dietary saturated for mono-saturated fat impairs insulin sensitivity in healthy men and women: The KANWU Study". *Diabetologia*, 44: 312–319.

World Health Organization. 1986. "Lifestyles and health". *Social Science Medicine*, 22: 117–124.

———. 1987. *Concepts of Health Behaviour Research.* Geneva: WHO.

———. 1994. *Prevention of Diabetes Mellitus: Report of a WHO Study Group.* Geneva: World Health Organisation (Tech Rep. Ser., no 844).

———. 1997. *The World Health Report 1997—Conquering suffering, enriching humanity.*

———. 2002. *The World Health Report 2002—Reducing Risks, Promoting Healthy Life.*

Yusuf, S., Hawken, S., Ôunpuu, S., Dans, T., Avezum, A., Lanas, F., McQueen, M., Budaj, A., Pais, P., Varigos, J. and Lisheng, L. on behalf of the INTER-HEART Study Investigators. 2004. "Effect of potentially modifiable risk factors associated with myocardial infarction in 52 countries (the INTERHEART study); case-control study". *Lancet*, 364 (9438): 937–952.

Chapter 6

Counselling in Primary Care

✍

◆ Andy CHEUNG, Samuel Y. S. WONG ◆

Introduction

As a family doctor, we never know who will walk through the door into the consultation room. Patients can be of any age group and present with almost any kind of problem. However illnesses of physical and/or psychological cause, when symptomatic, often present late in their development and thus are irreversible or are harder to deal with when diagnosed. Therefore among the various roles of a family doctor some of the most important ones are to be able to seek out these diseases in the early stages before they have a chance to develop into a full-blown infirmity, or ideally prevent them from happening in the first place.

For physical illnesses, primary prevention such as vaccinations, secondary prevention such as PAP smear screening, and tertiary prevention such as control of hypertension and diabetes are widely accepted practices. In psychological health, we tend to emphasise promoting nurturance throughout the family cycle from birth to enhance psychological well-being. We try to screen for psychological problems when patients present with very vague complaints or when they are proceeding to another stage in their family life cycle such as the beginning of parenthood. When patients are diagnosed with psychiatric problems, we would like them to adhere to treatment and follow up on them for early detection of relapse or recurrence. Unfortunately, many patients (sometimes doctors and society alike) do not treat psychological illnesses as they do with their physical ones and underestimate the importance to their health. Doctors thus need to be more aware and sensitive in providing psychological health care.

Important points for family doctors to remember during a medical consultation

- Keep "prevention" in mind and make the effort to improve psychological well-being of our patients as well as screening for (psychological) problems. This is especially true for those patients with any chronic illness. It is well-established that high incidences of depression occur in patients with diabetes mellitus, cardiovascular and respiratory diseases. Below is an example of a two question screening tool for major depression.

- Remind ourselves that symptoms and presentation of these problems may be subtle. If a patient's symptoms do not satisfy the *Diagnostic and Statistical Manual of Mental Disorders* (*DSM*, 4th Edition)/ *International Classification of Diseases* (*ICD*, 10th Edition) criteria of mental illness this does not necessarily mean that they do not require any form of intervention.

- It is not necessary to exclude all possible physical causes of the symptoms before we embark on mental health problems. Furthermore, mental health issues often co-exist with physical illness. Management can therefore be given in parallel as long as our assessment suggests that there are mental or psychological health issues.

- Patients usually present themselves to a family doctor when they are unwell. They may not be able to realise that this is due to psychological causes. These patients are unlikely to present themselves to a mental health worker of any sort. It may sometimes be difficult for them to accept that psychological or psychiatric factors are the only cause of their symptoms. Skills are required for the reattribution.

- Delay in treatment of psychological health problems may be as detrimental as delay in treatment of physical illnesses. For example, post-partum depression may be present in both father and mother and if left unattended would be detrimental to their marriage and their child's mental health (Coleman 2001).

- Whilst it is important to look after the psychological and physical health of our patients, family doctors should be equally concerned about their own psychological and physical health.

Screening Tool for Major Depression

1. During the past month have you been bothered by:
   • Feeling down, depressed or hopeless?
   • Little interest or pleasure in doing things?
2. Is this something with which you would like help?

Source: "Effect of the addition of a 'Help' question to two screening questions on specificity for diagnosis of depression in general practice: Diagnostic validity study". Arroll et al., *British Medical Journal*, 2005, 331: 884-886.

Sensitivity = 79% Specificity = 94%

Family doctors have many advantages in delivery of anticipatory care

• The patient knows you well as a doctor and a trusting relationship is often established even before any problem arises.

• With this trusting relationship, patients are more willing to talk about their problems, thus expediting the exploratory phase.

• Because of the previous encounters, family doctors know their patients well and will be able to notice something abnormal or unusual from non-verbal cues.

• For psychological problems, patients frequently approach a family doctor first and present themselves with physical symptoms.

• Patients usually talk about major life events with a family doctor. These are good opportunities for the doctor to screen for problems or to give anticipatory counselling.

• Sometimes care and support is the only thing that a patient wants in order to overcome the disruptions in their life.

What family doctors can achieve

• Based on epidemiology and clinical experience, one can identify people at risk and give appropriate counselling. An example is that young women (say under 16) who present to a clinic and admit sexual intercourse are more likely to report more psychological and (sexually unrelated) physical problems (Wong et al. 2004).

• Early detection of problems. For example, bereavement reactions such as people going through loss and grief, including loss of health, loss of relationships, loss of job etc. as well as the more obvious death of a friend, relative or loved one.

- Interventions. With some training, a family doctor can give supportive counselling, psycho-education, help patients with problem-solving skills, assertiveness skills or parenting skills. With more in-depth training and practice, one can use different counselling techniques and skills in different circumstances.

- Referral to other professionals if the problem is beyond their expertise or if time constraints prohibit.

- Following up on patients to ensure their well-being. For those diagnosed with psychiatric problems, early detection of relapses or recurrences is important.

Specific situations

Premarital counselling

People seldom doubt the necessity of screening for potential physical problems especially when these may affect the future generation. Contraceptive advice is welcomed and demanded. However potential marital tensions may pass unnoticed. The only person, apart from their relatives and friends, who may learn of the news is probably their family doctor. Furthermore there are many people who are reluctant and refuse to receive premarital counselling, with the excuse of a lack of time, or merely do not perceive it as necessary at a time when the couple appears to be very happy with their relationship. One of the roles of a family doctor is to bring up these issues and try to identify potential problems during the consultation.

Areas that can be covered

- If possible, observe the couple's means of communication and communication pattern. You may choose to ask specifically about who is the principal "talker" in their relationship and whether there is a high degree of indirect communication, i.e. "tend to hint at what they really mean, think or feel" and "tend to use 'it' or 'you' statements rather than 'I' statements" (Anderson and Sabatelli 2003). Attention is paid to statements such as: "We seldom talk about our feelings."; "We seldom quarrel because I won't challenge his opinion. I don't want to make him unhappy."

- Explore the family or origin of both sides, noting their family rules and values. It is worthwhile exploring how the man relates to his mother and how the woman relates to her father as the experiences may affect their current relationship with the opposite sex (Nichols and Schwartz 2001). Examples of statements deserving attention: "If my parents say yes, I would never say no."; "Sons are more important than daughters. In my family, men give orders and women have to comply."

- How does the couple handle conflicts? It would be useful to note whether one always avoid conflicts by constantly placating the other— if so was this what their parents did? Try to help them to be aware of potential differences and conflicts ahead of them and how to handle them when they happen. But at the same time point out that conflicts are healthy if handled appropriately viz. "Conflict is often necessary to encourage the changes and reorganizations that are required to make the relationship optimally responsive to both partners' needs" (Anderson and Sabatelli 2003).

- The individual values and expectations about the marriage including financial contribution, roles and expectations of each party even to the extent of task performance at home. These can be explored with the couple—is it reasonable, for example, that the wife does all the cleaning of the home, and the washing and looking after the children whilst the husband goes to work during the day and out with his friends in the evening whilst not contributing to the family home other than financially. The answer is surely that this depends on the couple—if they are both comfortable with this situation and it has no detrimental effect physically or emotionally on either party.

- Some people have unrealistic hopes that marriage will change their partner and invariably they will get extremely disappointed when it fails to do so. Statements such as the following should ring alarm bells to the doctor and should be discussed:
"I don't like his (certain behaviours). I hope he will change after we are married."
"She is too talkative and I hope that will change after the wedding."

- Explore power and boundary issues. Examples are: Who makes decisions and on what? Does one party expect the other to keep absolutely no secrets from them? Do they allow time or space for individual activities without involving the other half?

- Look at the closeness, intimacy and sexuality. Explore the mutual expectations on how to express closeness and intimacy and whether these behaviours are expected to be displayed exclusively to their partner. These are sensitive issues and care must be taken when we ask for this information.

- Enquire about spirituality as belonging to a different religion (or indeed being of different race/ethnicity) might create difficulties. Examples are: Is there any expectation that the other member will change their religion after marriage? If not, how are they going to handle the differences? What are the families' attitude to this situation and what effect will this have on the couple's relationship?

Other areas that potentially need further counselling

- They want to run away from a home that does not offer them love or security.
- They want somebody to support them financially.
- They solely want an extra pair of working hands at home.
- They want to show to their ex-girlfriend/ex-boyfriend who has left for someone else that they are capable of finding a replacement easily (somewhat of a revenge).
- Pregnancy is the reason for a marriage.
- Willingness to get married is because it is unfair to one party when they have already been together for many years. For example, patients may say, "I will feel guilty if I don't marry him/her."
- It seems that they are the only one available and your patient's family is putting pressure on them to get married as they are getting "old". The purpose of getting married is to satisfy parental expectation rather than their own needs.

Working with loss

Loss encompasses many different issues. For example, loss of health as in major illnesses; loss of relationships because of death or termination of relationships; or loss of jobs and thus self-esteem and control. Life transitions, including adaptation to new roles such as parenthood, inevitably include some loss. In these circumstances, patients may well present with physical symptoms such as headaches, back pain and so on. Although different stages of reaction are described when people face losses, these stages are non-discrete, may go back and forth throughout the process, and in some cases certain stages may never be entered at all.

Hypothesis and strategies

- People vary in the duration of and ability to adapt to change depending on the nature of the loss and individual's experience with loss.
- For bereavement, it is important to assess which part of the grief process the patient is experiencing:
  - ❖ Acceptance of the loss
  - ❖ Experiencing and expressing the pain and other emotions
  - ❖ Adjusting to an environment with the loss
  - ❖ Re-adjusting one's life into the external world and moving on
- When there is delayed grief (for example, under certain circumstances, a person is forced to go on with life as if nothing has happened during the loss and leave all feelings buried for years), re-experiencing the pain and expression of feelings may be necessary before the loss can be finally integrated.
- Complicated grief such as development of depression may require medical intervention such as the use of antidepressants as well as counselling.
- There may be gender differences in management of loss. According to the Dual Process Model by Stroebe et al., loss-oriented work with expression and sharing of feelings and emotions may be required more often for men as men usually try to suppress and not show their feelings. Restoration-focused work to learn new skills necessary to continue their life may be required more often for women as women usually indulge in emotions and ignore practical issues (Feltham and Horton 2000).

What a general practitioner can do when anticipating reactions to loss

- Normalise the reactions of our patients. Explain to the patient that what they are feeling or going through is normal and healthy. The emotional pain is often part of the healing process and if they do not go through it now, in the future when there is another life-event as there usually is, they will then have to deal with this issue again together with the new problem.

- Encourage the patient to identify their feelings and emotions. Reflect and ventilate, i.e. acknowledge those feelings to themselves and express them to others but always in a way that takes into account other people's feelings.

- Assess and understand the impact and meaning of the loss on the patient. The meaning of a loss is very individualised. For example, the loss of a person may to some people mean a loss of someone with whom they can share their hopes, visions and dreams, whilst for others it may mean a loss of security. The loss of health and loss of job may have impacts on one's sense of self and one's relationships with others. Remember that we must not be judgemental—imposing our own values or indeed our own feelings on our patients. For example, we may feel extremely sad if our parents pass away whilst our patients may not. We need to accept whatever reactions and responses are displayed by our patients. The main issue is that we want to know whether our patients are coping well or not. As discussed previously, support and understanding may be all that is required with some patients.

- Counsel our patients based on the impact and meaning of loss. Some of the meanings behind the emotions include:

Fear
  ❖ Insecurity about one's own future (for example, loss of financial support)
  ❖ Others may put the blame on them for the loss ("not being good enough")
  ❖ The impact of the loss on significant others (the loss of a sibling may affect their parents)

Anger/Disappointment
  ❖ On self, for not doing better
  ❖ On others, for not doing better
  ❖ The world, for being unfair

Sadness/Loneliness
  ❖ Lack of support after the loss

We should know our limitations and refer if necessary.

Doctor's emotional health

- Working with loss can be stressful for the helping professionals.

- Some may try to "cut-off" their own feelings and distance themselves from patients undergoing loss. However this may increase stress rather than decrease it as we need to admit our incompetence by avoidance. Doctors are no different from other people. If someone suppresses or denies their feelings these will still come out but in another guise. In the consultation the doctor may then appear frustrated or angry (if they have negative feelings) or over caring (if other emotions) instead of being neutral with the patient. Whereas if they acknowledge their own feelings they may be able to prevent these feelings from affecting the consultation.

- On the other hand, burnout may occur when our patients drag us into the loss experience, giving us a sense of helplessness.

- We must be aware of how we handle our own loss.

- Support from our peers and debriefing with colleagues are essential.

- Taking care of our own emotional health is of prime importance—it is all right to be ill and to feel stress. Doctors are not omnipotent beings!

Case example

Scenario

A 52-year-old clerk came to the clinic because of a small area of eczema over her right elbow. In addition, she complained of an occasional tingling sensation over both sides of the temporal region for the past three months. Each episode lasted for approximately 30 seconds. Sometimes there were several episodes within the same day, but she might be absolutely free of symptoms for several days. Her menopause was one and a half years ago. Her appetite was all right but her sleep was somewhat disturbed.

She was very worried about her younger sister who was diagnosed as having scleroderma and her condition was deteriorating. She felt unhappy because she was the only one in the family looking after her and the other siblings were not giving a helping hand. In addition, she was not happy at work because her new boss was very critical of her. She felt exhausted because she had to look after her sister and her own family, in addition to her job. Further exploration showed that her symptoms did not fit in any DSM IV criteria for any diagnosis.

She is married with two grown-up sons. Her relationship with her husband is good but they seldom share their feelings. There is no time for any recreation. Physical examination revealed nothing abnormal except for a very small patch of eczema over her right elbow.

What could be achieved in your consultation?

- Linking physical symptoms with mood and stress ("How has your mood been recently?", "If I say that your symptoms are due to stress/distress, do you think it is possible?").

- Explore how she is coping and narrow the focus ("What are the sources of stress?", "Which affect you most?").

- Explore the impact on her family and her husband's attitude to see if her husband is supportive. (If her husband is not supportive, what would she do? There will probably be guilt feelings whether she continues to look after her sister or leaves her alone.)

- Under these circumstances people tend to sacrifice themselves, neglecting their own physical, psychological and social health. They may not be aware of the detrimental effects until they are more severely affected.

- Let the patient be aware that she has done her best for her sister. She is probably unable to change what the other siblings do. So help her to accept and let go of her expectations of others.

- Stress the importance of looking after herself so that she is better able to look after her sister.

- Emphasise that her efforts have made a difference to her sister's life already and encourage her to accept her limitations.

- Nothing in life is perfect and "good enough" is what life is really about, i.e. set realistic goals for the patient.

Summary

- The presenting problem is a physical one. This probably serves as a ticket to consultation and the actual reason of the consultation is the more complex psychosocial problems.

- Stress can be managed more easily in a family medicine setting when the patients present themselves at an early stage. This also prevents further deterioration.

- When the symptoms are vague, we can work on the psychosocial issues after physical illness is excluded. This can be used as a therapeutic trial to show that the tingling sensation is probably due to her stress and distress.

- At such an early stage, patients are reluctant to seek help from counsellors. Stress and intense emotions not properly expressed can result in more long-term detrimental effects. Interpersonal relationships may be affected.

- Symptoms may be subtle and asking about our patient's mood is a key question in looking for possible psychological causes.

References

Anderson, S. A. and Sabatelli, R. M. 2003. *Family Interaction.* Boston: Allyn & Bacon, pp. 148–149, 168.

Coleman, W. L. 2001. *Supporting Parents. Family-focused Behavioral Pediatrics.* Philadelphia, PA: Lippincott Williams & Wilkins.

Feltham, C. and Horton, I. 2000. "Bereavement". In Feltham, C. and Horton, I., *Handbook of Counselling and Psychotherapy.* Thousand Oaks, CA: Sage, p. 445.

Nichols, M. P. and Schwartz, R. C. 2001. "Bowen family systems therapy". In Nichols, M. P. and Schwartz, R. C., *Family Therapy: Concepts and Methods* (5th edition). Boston: Allyn & Bacon, pp. 137–171.

Wong, W. C. W., Lee, A. and Tsang, K. K. 2004. "Correlates of sexual behaviors with health status and health perception in adolescents: A cross-sectional survey in schools in Hong Kong". *AIDS Patients Care and STDS*, 18 (8): 40–50.

Chapter 7

Psychological Issues in Primary Care

✑

◆ Samuel Y. S. WONG, Andy CHEUNG ◆

Introduction

In North America, it is estimated that between one-half and two-thirds of patients who consult their family doctor about a physical complaint are in fact seeking help to deal with emotional or psychological problems such as depression, anxiety or severe stress. Although no large population-based studies have been conducted in Hong Kong, cross-sectional surveys conducted locally showed that a significant proportion of patients seen by family doctors presented with psychiatric or functional problems (Chan et al. 2003). In a cross-sectional study conducted by Kessler et al. (2002), it was shown that general practitioners failed to diagnose up to half of the cases of depression or anxiety. In a subsequent study conducted by the same author, it was shown that although many patients with depression did not receive a diagnosis (61%) at a single consultation, most were given a diagnosis at subsequent consultations (40% of those not diagnosed) or recovered without a general practitioner's diagnosis. As a result, it seems that although depression may be missed in a single consultation, a large proportion will be diagnosed and dealt with in subsequent sessions by family doctors. For those who seek help, most are managed by their family doctors. When assessing a patient in primary care, doctors should consider psychological, social and physical factors on the mental health of their patient and the impact these factors may have on the choice of treatment of the mental health problem.

Psychological issues in primary care

Depression

According to some overseas studies, there are three main presentations of depression in a family medicine setting.

1. Presenting as unexplained somatic symptoms (but not necessarily psychosomatic as in *DSM* IV)
   - Physical symptoms such as chest pain, headache and numbness could be a part of depression
   - Patients may not think of themselves as being depressed as their symptoms are of a physical nature

2. With physical disease
   - Studies have shown that depression is associated with many chronic diseases, among which are cardiovascular diseases, COPD, cancer, arthritis, chronic pain osteoporosis (Wong et al. 2005) and diabetes
   - Depression often exacerbates pain and other physical discomforts (by reducing the individual's ability to withstand the pain/cope with the disability); treatment for depression may therefore improve physical symptoms

3. Presenting psychological symptoms
   - These patients present with psychological symptoms such as depressed mood, sleep disturbance, low self esteem and so forth, that fit the diagnostic criteria for depression

Anxiety

When there are both depressive and anxious symptoms and the main presenting symptoms are related to depression, the first priority should be to treat the depression since treatment for depression usually reduces anxiety. Furthermore, most antidepressants have anxiolytic effects. However with tricyclic antidepressants (TCA), the starting dose for treating anxiety is lower than that for treating depression (e.g. for depression the proven dose of a TCA is 100–125mg daily whilst for anxiety much lower doses from 10–50mg [depending on the TCA in question] are used. For selective serotonin reuptake inhibitors [SSRI] this dosage difference is not really relevant for the majority as the starting dose for anxiety and depression is the same).

There are several types of anxiety presentations that are commonly encountered in primary care:

1. Mixed anxio-depressive illness with predominantly anxiety symptoms

   Although anxiety symptoms may predominate, depression and anxiety usually co-exist. The predominant symptoms can vary over time, sometimes depending on the social environment and life events that the patients are experiencing.

2. Recurrent, intermittent brief episodes of panic or anxiety (Paroxysmal Anxiety Attacks)

   For these, you need to think about:
   - Panic disorder with or without agoraphobia
   - Exclude physical causes by history and physical examination, e.g. hyperthyroidism, phaeochromocytoma etc.
   - Consider drug induced, i.e. stopping benzodiazepines or antidepressants; too much stimulant (e.g. coffee, tea); illicit drug use such as amphetamines, cannabis, opiates
   - Consider hyperventilation as this could be an important perpetuating factor for continued anxiety

3. Longer lasting anxiety with over-arousal, irritability, poor concentration, poor sleeping and worry about several areas most of the time (Generalised Anxiety Disorder)
   - Generalised anxiety disorder with anxiety that lasts for more than 6 months with no single stressor

4. Anxiety triggered by external events
   - Specific phobias, e.g. agoraphobia, social phobia or needle phobia

Commonly, it is only after a few visits and sometimes extensive investigations that the patient will accept that their mind has some role to play in the physical symptoms that are so "real" to them. However if it is obvious that the symptoms are indeed psychological, it is often better to try and resist investigations and explain in detail why you are declining to investigate, as the mere referral for the tests tends to re-enforce the notion to the patient that they have a physical problem. In Chinese society, men may find it more difficult to surrender their well-being to a doctor or worse still, to be diagnosed as "mentally ill". It is at that moment that the communication skills and long-standing trust between the patient and the family doctor will have significant advantages. It is also a good idea not to use the term "mental illness" but to use alternative terms such as mental health problem to try and avoid societal stigmas.

Post traumatic stress disorder (PTSD)

PTSD is a delayed onset of anxiety/depressive type symptoms occurring after a severe and significant life event that persist for more than one month. It is thought that the individual's normal coping mechanism to such an event is overwhelmed. Examples might include rape, natural disasters such as a tsunami, seeing someone murdered and so on.

For most people who suffer such a traumatic event, there is a period of time during which they relive the event, which has obvious and understandable psychological consequences. However these usually subside. In PTSD the symptoms are very intense, debilitating and occur months after the event.

The prevalence of PTSD in the population is 2–3%. Those at greatest risk of developing PTSD are those with a pre-existing history of mental illness, the young and the elderly.

For PTSD to be diagnosed there are five criteria that have to be met:

1. The experience
   The person must have witnessed or experienced a significant threat (real or perceived) to their life

2. The re-experience
   The person must re-live all or part of that experience, e.g. flashbacks, nightmares, dreams, thoughts, feelings of guilt, phobias about specific daily routines

3. Avoidance
   The person persistently avoids the situations and/or those thoughts and emotions associated with or resembling the trauma

4. Physical symptoms of increased arousal
   Sleep disturbance, irritability, impaired memory and concentration, heightened "startle response", feelings of anxiety and inability to relax

5. Duration
   The symptoms last for more than one month

Co-morbidity

Anxiety/Depression and drug/alcohol misuse often co-exist.

Management strategies for psychological problems in family medicine

Psychological treatment

Family doctors can be ideally placed to act as effective counsellors, as the basis for counselling has already been established, i.e. trust. Moreover many patients who present with psychosocial problems may only need brief or short-term psychological interventions. For this the family doctor is well-placed. Others may need longer or more complex psychological therapy—for this referral to an appropriate professional or hospital department will be required.

Counselling does not mean simply giving information or advice. Instead, it is "the therapeutic process of helping a patient to explore the nature of his or her problem which facilitates insight and understanding". However most family doctors are not trained in this. Indeed, to be an effective counsellor, one has to explore one's own feelings. Many people find this potentially challenging (and family doctors are no exception). This is the commonest reason for "talking therapies" appearing to have failed. However it should be encouraged for all as it helps not only professionally but also in one's own life.

Counselling strategies in family medicine

For all treatment in family medicine, the patient's preference should be taken into account. Moreover history of relapse, response to treatment and patient's beliefs should also be considered in deciding the treatment approach.

Depression

Re-attrition. There are three stages:

* Feeling listened to and understood: patient feels doctor has understood their symptoms
    i. Take full history and get associated symptoms
    ii. Respond to mood cues and inquire about mood state
    iii. Explore social and family factors and situation
    iv. Understand health beliefs
    v. Perform a focused physical examination if indicated

    Although the outline above is simple, it should be noted that it may take several appointments in family medicine to conduct these counselling strategies. The beauty of being a family doctor is that we can get the patient back many times to complete this type of task and that in each consultation not only do we explore a bit more about the patient, but the patient also understands more about themselves and problem solving, i.e. the old adage "How do I know what I feel until I hear what I say?"

- The patient must reframe symptoms
  i.   Explain the results of physical examination and investigations
  ii. Acknowledge the reality of the patient's symptoms, i.e. "I can see that your pain is affecting your life" or "It must be difficult for you to feel such pain all the time"
  iii. Reframe the patient's complaint by reminding them of other symptoms and life events, and tentatively suggesting the link: "I wonder if, when you think about that you may feel depressed."
  iv. Give options and negotiate, e.g. "Let's see how we go and we may come back to this later."
- Making the link: how emotions can cause the symptoms
  i.   Explanation: linked to depression or anxiety
  ii. Demonstration: practical, i.e. think an anxious thought and feel the pulse; linked to life events, i.e. "In what situation are the symptoms most severe?"

Problem solving

- One of the components of Cognitive Behavioural Therapy
- Evidence of its effectiveness from randomised controlled clinical trials (Mynors-Wallis et al. 1995, 2000; Dowrick et al. 2000). It was found to be an effective, feasible and acceptable treatment for patients in family medicine (comparable to antidepressants in terms of efficacy)
- It can be particularly useful for those where antidepressants are not indicated (mild-moderate) or where patients prefer not to use non-pharmacological treatment after they have understood all the options
- As effective as antidepressants for mild depression. However it is more time-consuming (50 minutes per session and usually takes 6 sessions, although for some 12 sessions are needed). The stages are:
  i.   Ask the patient to identify their main problem
  ii. Ask them to think of possible solutions

iii. Suggest anything that you can think of, but has not been mentioned
iv. Prioritise the list; allow the patient to strike out impossible solutions
v. List advantages and disadvantages of each solution
vi. Settle on their preferred solution: break it down into steps
vii. They are to work on the first step of their preferred solution and report their progress to you

Cognitive behavioural strategies (CBS)

- Family doctors can provide specific and limited CBS to assist patients with depression, anxiety and somatisation disorders

- Teach patients' skills for enhancing more realistic interpretations of common life experiences and decreasing catastrophic interpretations

- Identify dysfunctional automatic thoughts/assumptions in patients and challenge their rational basis

- Give behavioural exercises such as graded exposure tasks which can be used to test the accuracy of various beliefs by gathering evidence for and against the old versus new beliefs

  Steps involved:
  i. Engage the patient
  ii. Identify unhelpful behavioural problems
  iii. Identify unhelpful thinking styles (or "habits")
  iv. Assist the patient to challenge negative unhelpful thinking in order to assist with emotional and behavioural change

Generalised anxiety disorder

- Benzodiazepines should not be used and medication generally should be used as a secondary treatment in the management of generalized anxiety disorder

- Antidepressant drugs, for example imipramine, clomipramine, paroxetine or venlafaxine, may be helpful. They do not lead to dependence or rebound symptoms, but can lead to withdrawal and should be tapered off gradually. However they can cause exacerbations of symptoms, thus all patients started on antidepressants should be reviewed 2 to 4 weeks after commencement

- Beta-blockers may help control physical symptoms such as tremor

- Cognitive behavioural therapy
- Explain links between worry and physical symptoms (psychoeducation)
- Encourage relaxation (e.g. muscle relaxation) or schedule pleasurable activities
- Physical exercise
- Practise problem solving

Panic disorder

- Common and treatable but usually by clinical psychologists or psychotherapists
- Regular use of benzodiazepines may lead to dependence and is likely to result in relapses of symptoms when discontinued. Thus it is best not to use them. One should encourage patients to face the situation without the use of benzodiazepines or alcohol by using alternative coping strategies as outlined above. However where the feared situation rarely occurs, short-term use of an antianxiety medication may be helpful, e.g. fear of flying
- If attacks are frequent and severe, or if the patient is significantly depressed, antidepressants may be helpful. Paroxetine and citalopram are licensed for treating panic disorder, although one should note that there may be slight worsening of symptoms initially and advice should be given to the patient to reduce activities for the week following the first prescriptions (see generalised anxiety disorder above)

Cognitive behavioural therapy (CBT)

- Self-help treatment (bibliotherapy—the use of written material to help people understand their psychological problems and learn ways to cope with them, i.e. CBT books)
- If possible, and if the patient is comfortable doing so, suggest the patient try not to avoid the stressor situation as avoidance behaviour tends to reinforce further fear and in the end may lead to agoraphobia or further problems
- Breathe slowly using the diaphragm and not chest wall muscles, i.e. practise relaxation techniques—over-breathing causes more panic

- "Self-talk technique"—"I am not going crazy/having a heart attack/ stroke, this is just a panic attack/symptoms from a panic attack, it will get better soon"
- Reduce coffee and tea or other caffeine-containing drinks, e.g. Coke
- Avoid alcohol and smoking

Phobias

- Use graded exposure (i.e. psychologist)
- Repeat mild exposure until no more fear (i.e. psychologist)
- Cognitive behavioural therapies (i.e. psychologist)
- Likely to need behavioural therapy (i.e. psychologist)

Non-pharmacological

- Encourage the patient and the family to discuss the event(s) and not to avoid such discussions
- Avoid the use of alcohol or other recreational drugs
- Explain to the patient and family about PTSD
- Encourage the patient not to persist with avoidance behaviours
- Consider referral for CBT especially in those whose symptoms are particularly debilitating
- Avoid pharmacological therapy except in severe cases or when there are significant co-existing mental health problems

Medical treatment

Depression

- There is no scientific evidence that people with only few or mild depressive symptoms respond to antidepressants
- For moderate/major depression, antidepressant medications across all drug classes have similar efficacy to psychological strategies such as cognitive behaviour therapy and problem solving techniques
- Patient preference, presence of associated problems in social or interpersonal relationships, family history and the experience and outcome of previous treatment(s) should be considered when deciding on treatment

- At present there is no evidence to suggest that any antidepressant is more effective than others. However their side-effect profiles differ and therefore some drugs will be more acceptable to particular patients than others

- Good management should include discussion with the patient about the nature of depression, its course, treatment options, side-effect profile of medication and likelihood of response to treatment. For dysthymia or chronic mild depression, TCA are equally effective compared to SSRI, e.g. fluoxetine and sertraline provided that a correct dose of TCA is used (i.e. 100–150 mg daily)

- The choice of antidepressants for major depression is influenced by five main factors: availability, side-effects, contra-indications (e.g. venlafaxine and cardiovascular disease), risk of suicidal intent and cost. Some have better effects for insomnia, e.g. mirtazapine and second line drugs such as venlafaxine

Side-effects

- In trials for comparing adverse effects and tolerance of antidepressants, SSRI appear to have slightly lower dropout rates when compared to first generation TCAs. However dropouts did not significantly differ for SSRI compared with second generation TCAs or tetracyclic antidepressants. Total dropout rates due to any reason appear to be no different between SSRI (31%) and TCA (33%) (Revicki et al. 1997)

- The common side-effects (> 10% in patients) in SSRI include dry mouth, headache, insomnia, nausea, diarrhoea and anxiety. For TCA, these are dry mouth, constipation, dizziness, blurred vision, tremors and headache. Various problems related to sexual dysfunction were reported in trials that include non-specific sexual problems, ejaculatory abnormality, decreased libido, male impotence, erectile dysfunction and anorgasmia

- These side-effects of antidepressants may settle within the first 2 weeks of treatment. As SSRI and venlafaxine may induce insomnia and anxiety during the initial stages of therapy, warn the patients and short-term benzodiazepines can be prescribed together for less than 2 weeks (though the latter are rarely needed especially if the patient is counselled about a possible initial worsening of symptoms)

Dosage

- Educate the patient: to take medication daily for at least 2–4 weeks for a therapeutic effect to be observed
- The need to continue treatment even when they feel better
- Not to stop medication without consulting a doctor
- Need to discuss the consequences of specific side-effects

Monitoring risk

- Patients started on antidepressants who are considered to present an increased suicide risk or are younger than 30 years should normally be seen after 1 week and frequently after as appropriate until the risk is reduced. In the UK it is now regarded as good practice to review all patients started on an SSRI after 2–4 weeks regardless of their initial suicidal status, i.e. even if no risk, as rarely some patients can become suicidal on these preparations

Duration of therapy

- A delay in onset of antidepressant response of at least 1–2 weeks after therapeutic dosage is reached
- The drug should be trialled for at least 4–6 weeks (4 weeks for no response and 6 weeks for partial response) after the therapeutic dose is reached before change of medication is considered
- As 35% of patients who discontinue antidepressant medication will experience relapse within 6 months, antidepressants should be continued for at least 6 months beyond initial recovery or improvement after a single episode of major depression to prevent a relapse within this period. Maintenance treatment has been shown to decrease the relapse rate for up to six months
- Long-term therapy (3–5 years) should be considered for those patients who have had 2 or more depressive episodes, 1 severe episode or a strong family history of recurrent depression

Ceasing antidepressants

- Withdrawal syndromes lasting a few weeks have been described with TCA, SSRI and venlafaxine, usually when the drugs have been taken for several months

- These symptoms include abdominal pain, nausea, vomiting, diarrhoea, insomnia, rhinorrhoea, light headedness and flu-like symptoms. Thus medication should be tapered off slowly over at least 4 weeks and longer for those with a shorter half-life, i.e. paroxetine

Generalised anxiety

- Medication management
    - ❖ Avoid the use of benzodiazepines
- Long-lasting anxiety
    - ❖ SSRI often helpful
    - ❖ Venlafaxine if cheaper SSRI ineffective and no cardiovascular contra-indication

Panic disorder

- SSRI and TCA antidepressants are both effective
- Need to continue for 6 months after response
- Taper off SSRI slowly
- Avoid benzodiazepines due to the possibility of dependence

Phobias

- Paroxetine has been approved for treating social phobia in Hong Kong. Antidepressants only if also moderately or severely depressed

Pharmacological treatment

- Consider a short course of a NON benzodiazepine hypnotic, e.g. zopiclone or diphenhydramine if there has been more than 4 consecutive nights of poor sleep
- Consider prescribing in the following circumstances:
    - ❖ For those with severe symptoms
    - ❖ Those whose PTSD lasts longer than 4 weeks
    - ❖ Those who decline CBT
    - ❖ If the wait for CBT is too long
    - ❖ If after CBT there has been no or minimal improvement
    - ❖ If there are significant co-existing symptoms of anxiety-depression

SSRIs are the drugs of choice. It is recommended starting with a low dose so as to avoid potential deterioration and reviewing the patient after a few weeks to ensure no decline, especially suicidal ideation. If at the review the drug is found to be tolerated, then increase the dose to that for depression. However there may be no obvious benefit for the first 8 weeks of treatment. If there are benefits by 3 months then continue for 15 months in total before considering gradual withdrawal.

Mental health services in Hong Kong

- Clinical psychologists (CPs) and counselling social workers from the Social Welfare Department, non-governmental organisations (NGOs) and family counselling organisations provide mental health services to the public

- CPs conduct psychological assessment and provide treatment for individual adults or children, couples, families and groups

- CPs treat depression, anxiety and stress, major mental disorders, learning disabilities, drug and substance abuse problems, marital/relationship problems and problems stemming from physical and sexual abuse

- Examples of NGOs that provide clinical psychological services:
  - ❖ Caritas Family Service
  - ❖ St James' Settlement
  - ❖ Christian Family Service Centre
  - ❖ Hong Kong Christian Service
  - ❖ Hong Kong Young Women's Christian Association
  - ❖ Hong Kong Sheung Kung Hui Tung Chung Integrated Services

Summary

- Identify psychological problems that require urgent referral or hospitalisation, e.g. suicidal patients

- Refer patients with psychological problems to psychiatrist when psychological problems do not improve or deteriorate with trial of 1–2 antidepressants at full therapeutic dose, depending on the physician's level of confidence and experience

- Refer patients to specialist mental health service for treatment resistant, recurrent, atypical and psychotic depression

- Importance of rapport and therapeutic relationships in the outcome of treatment

- Learn the basic skills of support counselling

- Know the cognitive behavioural strategies that can be applied for mild to moderate psychological problems

- Learn the duration, side-effects and indications for antidepressant use in depression, panic disorders and generalised anxiety

References

Chan, D. S. L., Wong, M. C. S. and Yuen, N. C. L. 2003. "The prevalence of functional disorders seen in family practice in Hong Kong". *The Hong Kong Practitioner*, 25: 413–418.

Dowrick, C., Dunn, G., Ayuso-Mateos, J. L., Dalgard, O. S., Page, H., Lehtinen, V., Casey, P., Wilkinson, C., Vazquez-Barquero, J. L. and Wilkinson, G. 2000. "Problem solving treatment and group psychoeducation for depression: Multicentre randomised controlled trial". *British Medical Journal*, 321: 1450.

Kessler, D., Bennewith, O., Lewis, G. and Sharp, D. 2002. "Detection of depression and anxiety in primary care: Follow up study". *British Medical Journal*, 325: 1016–1017.

Mynors-Wallis, L. M., Gath, D. H., Lloyd-Thomas, A. R. and Tomlinson, D. 1995. "Randomized controlled trial comparing problem solving treatment with amitriptyline and placebo for major depression in primary care". *British Medical Journal*, 310: 441–445.

Mynors-Wallis, L. M., Gath, D. H., Day, A. and Baker, R. 2000. "Randomized controlled trial of problem solving treatment, antidepressant medication, and combined treatment for major depression in primary care". *British Medical Journal*, 320: 26–30.

Revicki, D. A., Brown, R. E., Keller, M. B., Gonzales, J., Culpepper, L. and Hales, R. E. 1997. "Cost-effectiveness of newer antidepressants compared with tricyclic antidepressants in managed care settings". *Journal of Clinical Psychiatry*, 58 (2): 47–58.

WHO Guide to Mental Health in Primary Care (adapted for the UK from

Diagnostic and Management Guidelines for Mental Disorders in Primary Care: *ICD-10 Chapter V Primary Care Version*. Germany: Hogrefe & Huber Publishers, 1996).

Wong, S. Y. S., Lau, E. M. C., Woo, J., Lynn, H., Cummnings, S. R. and Orwoll, E. 2005. "Depression and bone mineral density: Is there a relationship in elderly Asian men. Results from Mr. Os Hong Kong, the first prospective cohort study of osteoporosis in Asian men". *Osteoporosis International*, 16: 610–615.

Chapter 8

Medico-legal Issues in Primary Care

◆ Nat YUEN, CHOI Kin ◆

Introduction

Over 5,000 years ago, the Hippocratic Oath set out the principles of medical ethics and introduced many concepts such as beneficence, confidentiality and justice. A number of updates, including the Declaration of Geneva, International Code of Medical Ethics and Declaration of Lisbon (World Medical Association 2006a, 2006b), have attempted to modernise it and to introduce new ideas that suit modern-day practices. For example, a doctor should "NOT permit considerations of religion, nationality, race, party politics or social standing" to intervene in their duty to patients (World Medical Association 2006a). The rights of patients and appropriate referrals were mentioned in the International Code of Medical Ethics, and the former was further elaborated and detailed in the Declaration of Lisbon. Some medical practices, e.g. termination of pregnancy was against the Hippocratic Oath but is now permitted under legislation in a restricted and controlled manner.

Many students find these concepts abstract and difficult to grasp. For example, according to the duties of a doctor registered with the General Medical Council (GMC, UK), doctors "have a duty to maintain a good standard of practice and care" (General Medical Council 2006). But what is a good standard of practice and care? The GMC tries to further define this by stating that a doctor must:

- Make the care of their patient their first concern
- Treat every patient politely and considerately
- Respect patients' dignity and respect their views

- Give patients information in a way they can understand
- Respect the rights of patients to be fully involved in decisions about their care

However how "polite" is polite? How much weight should a family doctor put on a patient's rights when it comes to decision-making? The clarification seems to beg more questions than answers. The author is aware of a complaint by a patient against a colleague who it was alleged, was too polite and indecisive. The complainant went on to say that the doctor was therefore not sincere and incompetent. Cases like this can be extremely demoralising to the professional.

This chapter aims to describe several features of ethics and law that may apply in family medicine which, taken together, make this discipline unique. Arguably, understanding the rights and obligations of a family doctor to their patients are the most important foundation stones for good and safe practices. We will then explore the laws and medical self-regulatory procedures that govern medical care and deal with complaints and medical litigations in Hong Kong.

Medical ethics that guide our practices in primary care

Family doctors provide primary care which, by its very nature, is comprehensive—seeing patients with any kind of query, symptom or problem. The care they provide is ongoing, providing the opportunity to gather a large amount of information about their patients and to develop a personal relationship over time. These features affect the nature of ethical issues presenting in family medicine in a number of ways.

Beneficence

The principle of beneficence requires doctors to act in the best interests of their patients. For family doctors who offer comprehensive, whole person care, acting beneficently involves the acceptance and integration of physical, psychological and social factors in the assessment and treatment of ill health. The patient's interests are more complex and broader in family medicine than in secondary or tertiary care. For example, a patient with a lacerated tendon in their index finger, sustained in a work-place accident, may present a straightforward technical problem to a plastic surgeon. The surgeon's responsibility is to repair the tendon competently and at most provide a report to support a future claim by the patient. However for the family doctor, the problem may be more complex. There are many factors which may impact upon this person's recovery including their relations with the employers, the financial costs of the injury, the impact upon future employment and the demands of their family. Acting in the best interests of this patient requires skilful consideration of all of these factors, which may well influence their recovery. Medical expertise is necessary to act for the patient's benefit in family medicine, but medical expertise contributes a smaller proportion of the overall expertise required. The patient's own experience is also crucial in determining the best action.

As we have seen, family doctors have a significant role in health promotion and education. Health promotion and preventive care raise a number of ethical issues, as these activities do not occur in response to requests for medical care but are more often initiated by the doctors themselves. For example, good family medicine requires preventive care such as the prevention of coronary heart disease, cerebrovascular accident and cancer. However it is important to avoid a coercive attitude about patients' risk factors, particularly when a doctor advises their patients to change their lifestyle, such as renunciation of favourite foods, alterations to patterns of socialisation, changes in leisure activities and so on. These situations raise interesting questions about the boundaries of beneficence, especially when the benefits of such changes are hard to predict.

Respect for autonomy

Medical care has rapidly moved away from a paternalistic approach towards patient autonomy. However some "patient-centred" doctors have gone beyond allowing patients to participate in decision-making, and in some extreme cases force them to decide on their own and avoid making recommendations to them. This is regarded as the "Independent Choice Model". The patients have independence and control whilst the doctors serve as passive informers. Here the doctors are detached and abdicate the responsibility to patients. This can potentially do harm to the patient-doctor relationship. On the other hand, the "Enhanced Autonomy Model" allows more sharing between doctors and patients on knowledge and expertise. The doctor serves as an active guide, which enhances the relationship of trust. Patients and doctors collaborate with each other and so share the joint responsibility for patient outcome. Issues of autonomy do not revolve around single instances of informed consent to complex or dangerous procedures. Patients should be informed about the therapeutic possibilities and their odds of success. In addition, patients' values and own recommendations are to be explored as the basis of their management plan. To enhance the patients' autonomy, open dialogue is essential. This includes active listening, honest sharing of perspectives, suspension of judgement and genuine concern about the patients' best interests. Studies have shown that enhanced support of patient autonomy has been associated with better outcomes in substance abuse treatment, weight reduction and adherence to treatment regime.

In family medicine, there is the opportunity to understand the circumstances of the patient and to recognise the impact of ill health upon that person's life. Determining the amount of information to be shared with patients can be difficult, especially as there is considerable time pressure on consultations. This difficulty is offset by the ongoing nature of family medicine where it is possible to provide information over time and to help patients to build up their understanding of their health problems. This provides the opportunity to empower patients and to help them achieve greater autonomy in managing their health care. The central philosophy of autonomy is respect for the patient as a person. The personal knowledge that family doctors have of their patients means that they can tailor information to particular patients, recognising the differences between individuals in their desire for information.

Generally speaking, patient autonomy induces impacts at different levels. At the patients' level they can be more informed about treatment options so that a more informed decision can be made. Conversely, in this informative world, where patients have easy access to medical information, much uncertainty and sometimes more conflicts or misunderstanding may be created whilst in others this may facilitate more effective communication between the doctor and the patient. From the doctors' perspective, some doctors may think that they could be safeguarded against lawsuits because the management plan is agreed by both parties. Nevertheless doctors have to be aware of the information given to patients, their understanding and the "true" choice by patients in which beneficence is seriously considered. As far as social level is concerned, enhanced patient autonomy can balance the power structure between patients and doctors.

The doctor-patient relationship

The continuing nature of the care offered by family doctors has ethical dimensions. Care is not limited to specific episodes of illness or courses of treatment but continues through health and illness, both acute and chronic.

This long-term commitment has some important consequences, particularly the growth of strong relationships between patients and their doctors. Within such relationships, family doctors accumulate large amounts of personal information about patients, including their preferences for types of therapies, their responses to illness, their supports and strengths and weaknesses. Similarly, patients also build up a considerable amount of knowledge about their doctors: knowledge about their views on health and illness, propensity to investigate, refer or prescribe, and ways of communicating. The cornerstone to the success of these relationships is trust, which may be built up over time. There are a number of ways in which trust can operate in the doctor-patient relationship. First, family doctors have a responsibility to be trustworthy in their medical knowledge and competence, and trustworthy in their goodwill towards their patients. In addition, they need to trust their patients, not only in terms of their veracity and commitment to co-operate with care, but also to have trust in patients' capacities to understand information and to make decisions. Patients have similar responsibilities— to be trustworthy in their motives for seeking medical advice and in their intentions to cooperate with care. The presence of trust eases communication and the process of medical care, fostering beneficence without paternalism and respect for autonomy without contractual or consumerist overtones. In the context of a trusting relationship, it is easier to deal with crises and to accommodate the pressures which arise in any ongoing relationship. Long-term commitment of this kind may be seen as a form of constancy; a promise to remain with the patient even when the medical profession has little to offer.

Justice

Family doctors serve as gatekeepers, authorising access to more expensive specialist care and also co-ordinating such care. In this gatekeeping role, family doctors are potentially faced with issues of justice and conflicts between trying to obtain optimal care for individual patients whilst operating within a financially finite system. Family doctors are traditionally strong advocates for their patients, but at the same time they (particularly those working in the public sector) have to be aware of their social responsibilities. This requires exercising judgement about the need for and timing of referrals. Sometimes a patient may benefit from the reassurance of a negative investigation such as an x-ray; this benefit must be weighed up against the cost of the investigation and the needs of other patients.

Communication

Family doctors are situated at the centre of a complex web of communications with different parties. Referring patients to secondary care requires accurate communication of confidential materials. It is important to make sure that patients understand that relevant information will be shared between specialists and family doctors.

From time to time, doctors are called upon by their patients to explain results or decisions made by other doctors. These activities are facilitated by cordial relationships between primary and secondary care, with recognition of the constraints such as consideration of the mental state of the patient and other resources limitation in the public sector operating upon all parties.

Family doctors are part of the primary health care team, sharing responsibility for health care with other professionals and support staff. Courtesy and consideration, as well as respect for the skills of others, eases these relationships and provides an appropriate atmosphere for optimal patient care.

Confidentiality

Maintaining patient confidentiality is a key ethical issue by family doctors. Confidentiality can be difficult, not only because family doctors work as part of a primary health care team but also because they treat families rather than individual patients. Parents may request confidential information about a child, demanding loyalty from the doctor in a way which compromises professional integrity. One partner with a sexually transmitted infection may ask for the other partner to be treated without their knowledge, or the doctor may be asked to withhold information about life threatening illnesses such as HIV. A family doctor may be aware of a patient's health problem which should disqualify them from driving, such as epilepsy or poor vision. The GMC provides detailed information on dealing with situations such as these, when concern about the safety of others may override confidentiality. (See also the section on Professional Code and Conduct from the Medical Council of Hong Kong: www.hkmc .org.hk.)

Family doctors provide medical certificates and other reports which can raise issues of confidentiality. It is important to make sure that patients understand the implications of divulging health information to third parties, especially when this information may hinder a patient's application for life insurance or disability benefits. One specific situation in Hong Kong is foreign domestic maids where they work and live often under close supervision with their health expenses being paid for by their employers. In addition there are sometimes language barriers. Thus doctors may be under more pressure to bypass the strict rule of confidentiality. Confidentiality may also be compromised by requests for information about patients made by researchers. The lists of patients registered with family doctors are valuable sources of information for epidemiologists and other primary care researchers. However there are strict regulations, including the Data Protection Act 1998 and Professional Code and Conduct, governing access to this information. Any requests for patient information require doctors to seek consent from the patient, to hide the patient's identity in the data provided where possible and to keep disclosures to the minimum.

Consent

Doctors have a duty of care across the continuum of diagnosis, treatment and information disclosure. Sometimes doctors encounter a dilemma when the patient's dutiful relatives ask them not to unveil the diagnosis to the patient. It is in fact the obligation of doctors to inform the patient so that consent for treatment can be obtained. Relatives can only be considered in reference to a patient's wishes but they can never decide for the patient.

Informed consent is a process of communication between a patient and a doctor that results in the patient's authorization or agreement to undergo a specific medical intervention. Consent is part of quality care as well as a legal requirement. Medical treatment can only be provided on the basis of the patient's informed consent, or withdrawn on the basis of the patient's informed refusal. Treatment without consent may be justified in an emergency. In that case, doctors should only give treatment that is urgent and crucial in the best interests of the patient. It can also be applied to the situation where a mentally competent adult is unconscious or where they are conscious but unable to communicate a decision. A doctor can lawfully operate on or give treatment to adult patients who are temporarily incapable without consent in order to preserve life or ensure improvement or prevent deterioration.

Certain important information should be included in a proper consent form (Table 8.1). A valid consent process is indeed crucial whenever it is encountered during a consultation. Patients are then more compliant and willing to share the responsibility. They are more realistic about the

Table 8.1 Checklist for a proper consent form

• name of operation	• special precautions required post-operation
• nature of proposed treatment	
• what the operation involves	• benefits of treatment
• other treatment options or alternatives	• limitations of treatment
• potential complications	• success rate of operation
• risks of operation	• what happens on admission
• risk of no treatment	• how patient will feel after treatment

possible outcomes of treatment and in turn the risk of litigation of doctors will be reduced. As a result, the doctor-patient relationship is improved. The key to achieving this process is good communication skills. Doctors who fail to establish good relationships with patients will endanger trust and confidence. Those who spend time to explain are less likely to be subjects of complaints. Thus it is advisable that doctors spend some time on clarifying the understanding of patients and encouraging them to raise queries and concerns.

Further issues

The pharmaceutical industry cultivates relationships with community doctors through practice visits by pharmaceutical representatives. It is unethical to accept gifts or inducements from sales representatives. Hospitality in the form of sponsorship of educational meetings by pharmaceutical companies is common. Doctors must decide individually whether or not they are compromised by accepting such hospitality. In addition, the pharmaceutical industry frequently performs research in primary care settings and may offer financial incentives to doctors for enrolling patients in trials. Full disclosure of financial incentives is crucial when enrolling patients, as is review of research by a local research ethics committee.

Sometimes patients may make requests about which family doctors feel uncomfortable, such as requests for "sick notes" with little apparent evidence of ill health. These situations require conscientious deliberation and discussion with patients. Doctors have a responsibility to only sign statements they believe to be true. The population seen by family doctors in Hong Kong can be culturally varied, with people from many different ethnic backgrounds. Learning about and respecting the diverse perspectives of others is a crucial part of providing good primary care. The interactions between cultures and structural influences on health care involving different disadvantaged groups such as sex workers or the mentally retarded can constitute major barriers to health care, thus requiring doctors to make every effort to provide culturally appropriate medical care.

Case Study 1 Issuing untrue or misleading medical certificates

Scenario

Dr. O was charged with 12 disciplinary offences, namely that on 12 occasions in the period between August 1997 to September 1998, Dr. O issued retrospective and untrue sick leave certificates to a number of patients.

The Medical Council's findings

The Legal Officer produced movement records from Immigration Department to prove that a certain named patient was not in Hong Kong on the dates of the sick leave certificates and it was impossible for Dr. O to have examined the patient on the aforementioned dates.

The Medical Council's ruling

The Council pointed out that medical practitioners are required to issue reports and certificates on the assumption that the truth of the certificates can be accepted without question. The Council always considers issuing untrue certificates a serious offence. The council ordered that the name of Dr. O should be removed from the General Register for a period of 1 year.

Case Study 2 Issuing untrue or misleading medical certificates

Scenario

On June 2003, a doctor was charged with the following disciplinary offences: "issued and signed three sick leave certificates by using another registered medical practitioner's chop". The defendant doctor admitted that he was the author of the certificates in question. His explanation was that he was a locum doctor at the other doctor's clinic and used his stationery. The sick leave certificates were stamped with the other doctor's name chop by the clinic staff. The defendant made an inadvertent administrative error in signing those certificates on the other doctor's name chop.

The Medical Council's findings

The Council was satisfied that the facts of the charges were proved and found the defendant guilty as charged. The penalties for issue of improper sick leave certificates vary from a warning letter to removal from the register. Doctors are warned to be extremely careful about their sick leave forms and should keep them under lock and key to avoid their being stolen by clinic staff for improper usage.

Laws of Hong Kong in relation to medical practice

In Hong Kong, the laws on the practice of medicine are governed by the Medical Registration Ordinance, Chapter 161, and the Medical Practitioners (Registration and Disciplinary Procedure) Regulations. The legislation covers the structure and activities of the Hong Kong Medical Council, which is also the watchdog for professional discipline.

The Medical Council of Hong Kong is composed of representatives from the Department of Health (2), the University of Hong Kong (2), The Chinese University of Hong Kong (2), the Hospital Authority (2), the Hong Kong Academy of Medicine (2) and the Hong Kong Medical Association (7), as well as 7 elected medical professionals and 4 lay persons. It has 5 standing committees, namely:

• The Licentiate Committee

• The Education and Accreditation Committee

• The Ethics Committee

• The Preliminary Investigation Committee

• The Health Committee

Its main functions are to: (1) Register, accredit and licentiate examinations; (2) Consider ethical and health issues of medical practitioners; and (3) Deal with disciplinary matters. Based on the types and severity of offences committed, the Council may take one or more actions against offending medical practitioners by issuing a warning letter, publicising the matter in the Gazette, referring the case to the Health Committee, issuing a reprimand and suspension or even removal of the registration from the General Register.

How does The Medical Council deal with complaints?

Once a complaint is filed, it will go to the Preliminary Investigation Committee (PIC) which will decide if there is a case for further investigation. It can be a convicted case from the court or a complaint filed by the general public.

Other laws of Hong Kong relevant to family doctors

To a lesser extent, the Pharmacy and Poisons Ordinance and Regulations, Chapter 138, Dangerous Drugs Ordinance, Chapter 134, and Offences Against The Person Ordinance, Chapter 212, of Hong Kong are also involved.

Case Study 3   Failure to note the Dangerous Drug Ordinance

Scenario

On 14 July 2004, a doctor was charged with the following disciplinary offence:

"That he, being a registered medical practitioner, was convicted at the North Kowloon Magistrates Court on 19 June, 2003 of 47 offences punishable with imprisonment, namely 47 counts of failing to keep proper record of dangerous drugs, contrary to Regulations 5(1)(a) and 5(7) of the Dangerous Drugs Regulations, made under the Dangerous Drugs Ordinance, Chap. 134, Laws of Hong Kong."

The Medical Council's findings

The Council noted that the case involved breach of the statutory duty in three aspects:

- The identity card numbers of all the patients to whom the drugs were supplied were missing from the records
- There were unauthorised alterations to 40 out of the 47 records
- There were serious discrepancies between the dangerous drugs seized and the balances recorded in the registers of drugs

In mitigation, the defence claimed that it was a technical breach of the law. The Council did not accept the mitigation. It pointed out that the requirement to maintain proper records of all dangerous drugs in strict accordance with the statutory forms under the Dangerous Drugs Regulations is set out in detail in paragraph 11.2 of the Professional Code and Conduct, and the Form of Register under the Dangerous Drug Regulations is reproduced in Appendix C of the Code. All registered practitioners should be well aware of what is required of them under the law.

The Council commented that "we note that some of the drugs in question were addictive drugs, liable to abuse, and the quantity of drugs involved in the discrepancies were extraordinarily large. Registered medical practitioners are given the privilege to possess and supply dangerous drugs, and with the privilege comes a heavy responsibility to ensure that the drugs are carefully controlled and accounted for so as to prevent the drugs from falling into the wrong hands. It is no mitigation that the defendant was not fully aware of the responsibility, nor to say that the duty was carried out carelessly by the nurses on his behalf."

All registered doctors are advised to fill in and check their own registers and not to leave it to their staff. Registered doctors alone are responsible for the keeping of the register and it is no mitigation to put the blame on the clinic staff, as demonstrated in the previous example.

Medical negligence

People in the community must be able to trust their doctors with their sickness and well-being. In order to justify that trust, doctors have a duty and honour to maintain a good and ethical standard of practice and care to their patients and to demonstrate respect for human life. Once that contractual relationship is established but the doctor fails to provide a good standard of care and harm (be it physical or psychological or both) results due to their action or lack of action, a case of medical negligence is found. The section "the nature of medicine" from the booklet published by the Medical Council is worthy of consideration:

"In medicine, a given set of symptoms may for instance indicate not one, but several possible diagnoses. There are generally accepted medical methods of attempting to arrive at the correct diagnosis and appropriate treatment. Providing a doctor has adopted an acceptable standard of medical practice, the fact that an incorrect diagnosis has been made is not, of itself, an indication of professional misconduct. This is particularly so if the symptoms presented by the patient fit the diagnosis. Similarly, an unsatisfactory outcome of a surgical procedure is not necessarily an indication of incompetence or negligence on the part of the doctor. Whilst there are general similarities in body structure and the way human body's system work, there are sufficient variations in these areas to cause unforeseen or unforeseeable problems in some patients even with the best of surgical or medical expertise being applied. Different methods of treatments may cause different results. However, there are some guidelines set out in the 'Professional Code and Conduct' for doctors to follow. It is therefore advisable for doctors to read through the guidelines carefully thereby avoiding the danger of inadvertently transgressing accepted codes of professional ethical behaviour, which may lead to disciplinary action by the Medical Council."

Case Study 4   Failure to refer or treat

Scenario

A doctor was charged with failing "to refer the patient to a hospital or an appropriate medical institution for urgent and appropriate treatment" after "having diagnosed that the patient was suffering from heart disease" "where such referral would be necessary in the circumstances of the case".

On 27 April, 2001, the defendant conducted an electro-cardiogram (ECG) examination on the patient. On the basis of the ECG, she diagnosed that the patient was suffering from heart disease and wrote a referral letter for the patient to be seen by a cardiologist. On 28 April, 2001, the patient went to the cardiologist for consultation and collapsed in the cardiologist's office. The patient was immediately taken to hospital by ambulance and she died shortly afterwards.

The defendant doctor admitted that she made an error in failing to recognise from the ECG that the patient was suffering from acute myocardial infarction. The defence however contended that a general practitioner in the defendant's position who had little exposure to ECG could understandably make such mistakes, and the mistake was excusable.

An expert in family medicine was called to give evidence. He was of the opinion that the ECG of the patient clearly indicated acute myocardial infarction and any competent medical practitioner including a general practitioner should be able to diagnose the condition from the ECG. He testified that such knowledge on the interpretation of ECG would be acquired in the course of a medical practitioner's undergraduate teaching. He gave evidence that acute myocardial infarction required immediate referral of the patient to a hospital for urgent treatment.

The Medical Council's findings

The Council accepted the expert's evidence that any registered medical practitioner should have been able to make a proper diagnosis, based on the ECG of the patient, that the patient was suffering from acute myocardial infarction which required her immediate referral for urgent treatment. In this regard the Council was satisfied that the defendant had fallen below the standard expected among registered medical practitioners. The Council was satisfied that this amounted to misconduct in a professional respect. It therefore found the defendant guilty as charged.

The Medical Council's order

The Council ordered that the defendant be reprimanded; such an order to be suspended for the period of two years subject to the condition that she undergoes within the suspension period such continued medical education as approved by the Medical Council, equivalent to a certificate course in family medicine.

Case Study 5   Misdiagnosis

Scenario

A 32-year-old flight attendant contracted cerebral malaria in South Africa and died on 14 December, 2001. The attending doctor mistakenly diagnosed the case as influenza. The coroner's court decided on a verdict of "death by natural causes to which neglect contributed". The verdict was later rescinded by the High Court judge who stated that the doctor's diagnosis and treatment did not contribute to her death. Since this case and the subsequent Severe Acute Respiratory Syndrome (SARS) epidemic and bird flu scare, all doctors should be more vigilant in asking about patients' travelling histories if they present with a fever.

Claim procedures in medical negligence

Claims are rarely made soon after an adverse incident has occurred. There can be long delays between an incident and subsequent challenge: even after death! The period within which a patient may make a negligence claim usually dates from the time the patient becomes aware that they have suffered harm. Moreover in the case of minors, the limit is usually extended to the age of majority, and where permanent disability has been caused or in cases of mental incompetence, the period may be indefinite.

The following table shows a typical pattern for the percentage of claims by number reported each year in respect of medical accidents occurring in 1997. By 2006, 5% of claims still have not been resolved and it is often these late claims that involve brain-damaged children and are consequently the higher value ones.

Table 8.2 Percentage of medical accident claims per year

Year claim reported	1997	1998	1999	2000	2001	2002	2003	2004	2005	2006
% reported (per year)	8	18	15	12	12	10	8	6	4	2
% reported (cumulative)	8	26	41	53	65	75	83	89	93	95

Although it is not illegal to practise in Hong Kong without medical indemnity insurance, it is strongly advisable to have such insurance. When a member requires more assistance than just telephone advice, an insurer such as the Medical Protection Society (MPS) will open a file on a particular case. The MPS defines a case as a claim whenever there is a demand for compensation for harm caused by an adverse incident (irrespective of any negligence or harm caused). A lawyer is not necessarily involved and many will not end up in court, but the intention by the patient or relative is the same. All other files are called "non-claims files" but some, in time, may become claims. For example, a member may report an adverse incident to the MPS and at that time there is no intention by the patient to sue, but it is possible that they decide several years later to pursue an action against the doctor.

What can doctors do to minimise the risk of complaints/ litigation?

Medical negligence unfortunately is increasing and it is likely to increase further in the near future. The following figures show the extent of medical negligence in Hong Kong:

- There are currently over 200 ongoing claims or reported matters that could become claims against MPS members in Hong Kong

- 20% have an estimate of over HK$1,000,000 with more than a dozen with estimates over HK$10,000,000

- MPS estimated that the average claim size of claims arising from incidents in 2005 will be 6.5% higher than the previous year and the claims frequency 27% higher

Whether it is a doctor's fault or not, any legal proceedings will be very stressful for the doctor concerned. Thus the best way is to avoid it happening in the first place. All doctors are well-advised by the Medical Council to read through the "Professional Code and Conduct" issued to all registered medical practitioners. By acquainting themselves thoroughly with its contents, doctors may be able to avoid the danger of inadvertently transgressing the accepted codes of ethical professional conduct, which may lead to disciplinary action by the Council.

The Medical Protection Society has advised that many complaints/ litigation in fact arose out of misunderstanding and communication breakdown between the patient and the doctor. One of its publications, "A smile a day keeps the lawyers away", outlines "the importance of effective communication in preventing litigation" (Hegan 2004). The article also describes why patients sue their doctors and what patients want when they sue. It is indeed an article worth reading.

References

General Medical Council. Retrieved 17 January, 2006, from http://www.gmc-uk.org/.

Medical Council of Hong Kong. 1998. *How the Medical Council Deals with Complaints.*

Hegan, T. J. 2004. "A smile a day keeps the lawyers away". *Melta Medical Journal*, 16 (2): 42–45.

World Medical Association. 2006a. "Declaration of Geneva". Retrieved 17 January, 2006, from http://www.wma.net/e/policy/c8.htm.

———. 2006b. "Declaration of Lisbon". Retrieved 17 January, 2006, from http:// www.wma.net/e/policy/l4.htm.

Chapter 9

Partnership with NGOs in Health Care

✑

◆ Albert LEE ◆

Family doctors provide comprehensive and whole person care. Not only do they act as an initial contact, they are also the most important resource persons for their patients. However family doctors cannot solve all the problems of their patients because some problems are beyond the boundary of the family medicine clinics due to constraints on time, facilities and/or skills. Therefore family doctors should fully collaborate with other professionals (in both health and social sectors) in investigation and resolution of patients' problems. One of the skills of the family doctor is to work across clinical boundaries. Family doctors can bring in extra community resources, such as non-governmental organisations (NGOs), in delivering holistic care to their patients.

With the increase in chronic illnesses, in part due to an ageing population, shifting health care towards the community provides one of the greatest potential for cost-effective mode of delivery. However the problems faced by patients with chronic diseases are not always ameliorable by the curative approach of much of modern medicine. The same applies to care of the elderly. Chronically ill patients and their families require a great deal of support in the community. As already discussed elsewhere in this book, illness has significant impacts on psycho social and physical well-being, including daily activities, as well as on the family and carers. Community-based rehabilitation enhances the quality of life of these patients and their families through provision of psychosocial rehabilitation, promotion of self-help and mutual support, patient empowerment, self-care, training for the carers, mobilisation and training of volunteers.

If we take stroke as an example, family doctors will play an important role in ameliorating the potential risk factors and monitoring the patient's condition. However a stroke patient needs to be empowered to carry out their usual daily activities. Their family members and carers have to be trained and supported in order that they can look after and meet the needs of the stroke patient in the community. The disease has strong impacts on the psychosocial well-being of the patient. Patients and family members may need counselling from time to time to cope with the change of health status and the disability resulting from their illness. Self-help and peer support are very useful for patients and family members, enabling them to gain experience in self management of the illness. Apart from the professionals, lay volunteers can either be trained as peer counsellors in psychosocial rehabilitation or provide additional home help to relieve the burden on the family members. They can also help to launch community programmes for the patients and families to minimise their roles as ill persons and help them to re-integrate with their community.

In Hong Kong, an NGO called Community Rehabilitation Network (CRN) has developed an innovative approach in providing community-based rehabilitation services "by making use of resources available in the community to empower the patients and/or the carers in maintaining their usual functional status as far as possible to minimise dependency". The Department of Community and Family Medicine of The Chinese University of Hong Kong was commissioned to conduct a consultancy study in 1998 to review the existing CRN services and to make recommendations for its future development, in particular interfacing strategies with other service providers (Lee et al. 1999). On the whole, the study found that the services provided by CRN were effective and able to meet the needs of most chronically ill patients. However the scope of the service provided was too broad, which could lead to problems of lack of focus and depth. Thus the CRN was advised to concentrate on its strengths: counselling, therapeutic aspects of group activities, networking and liaison, and patient-empowerment intervention. These kinds of services would supplement the services provided by family doctors in the management of patients with chronic illnesses, especially those doctors in solo practice who are often too pressurised to be able to spend the necessary time with these patients. If family doctors have access to those same services, and the community-based rehabilitation services, such as CRN have already had access to the expertise of family doctors in the clinical setting of chronic illness management, the two types of services would have a synergistic effect in maintaining or indeed improving the care of patients in the long run. Therefore the consultancy study also recommended that the CRN should be more actively involved with family doctors in community rehabilitation, as they could more effectively act as good gatekeepers to the hospitals. Family doctors can also provide frontline medical backup to the CRN in the community, with the specialists providing second line backup. Moreover the doctors in the private sector, including the private hospitals, should be made aware of the existence of CRN services. The CRN should be able to fill the service gap for patients not being treated by the public hospitals. No government provides all services without gaps and the NGOs can fill in those gaps left over by the government's financial support.

Another model is, for example, for a family doctor to establish an outreach clinic with an NGO that works for marginalised or vulnerable groups of society, arguably the social responsibility of family doctors. Voluntary clinical sessions in the form of "well women/well men clinics" have been set up on a part-time basis at NGO sites. A decision analysis comparing an outreach clinic to the usual medical care in Hong Kong found that the outreach approach appeared to be less costly and more effective in preventing gonorrhoea and chlamydia transmission between female sex workers and their clients (You and Wong 2005). There is no medico-legal implication in operating such a clinic so long as it is run by a registered medical practitioner and provides a good standard of practice. Medical indemnity insurance is usually covered by the existing policy at no extra cost. Work in this area tends to be very satisfactory, but NGOs may have different agenda from the medical ones.

A Charter for Family Medicine in Europe—WHO Regional Office stated that, by the year 2000, all member states should meet basic needs by providing services on health promotion, curative, rehabilitation and supporting services, and supporting self-help activities for individuals, families and groups. This led to the concept of "New Family Medicine" being described as the science and art of providing community-based personalised health services to patients through curative and preventive medicine; looking for partnership in the community to form healthy alliances in promoting positive health; and working together in determining the health needs and setting the priority area in the catchment area (Lee 2000). This new era would motivate family doctors to move beyond the clinic walls into the community and participate actively in community affairs. Family doctors need to take a strong initiative in forming healthy alliances so that they can have a greater influence on health policy formulation. NGOs can play an important role in this.

If family doctors want to function effectively as gatekeepers to secondary care, and to become the most important first contact of patients in need of medical assistance and advice, they must work in a well-integrated primary healthcare system. However not all countries provide a well-structured primary healthcare system and fragmentation of services does occur all the time. Family doctors working together with NGOs and the government services can establish a very good district-based platform to facilitate collaboration among health professionals and also other professionals in the shared care of patients.

Many organisations provide an updated profile of NGOs in different districts (see Appendix). Family doctors can explore the different roles played by the NGOs in their catchment areas and should be encouraged to establish their own network in their district in liaison with NGOs well before they are confronted with a needy case. This will avoid unnecessary duplication of services and add synergy to the healthcare delivery system.

References

Lee, S. H., Lee, A., To, C. Y., Ho, K. F., Phua, K. H. and Tsang, K. K. 1999. *Consultancy Report to Hong Kong SAR Government on Evaluation of Community Based Rehabilitation Network.* Department of Community and Family Medicine, The Chinese University of Hong Kong.

Lee, A. 2000. "Public health and personal health: The concept of new family medicine and re-orientation of primary health care to face the challenges in the 21st century". *Asia Pacific Journal of Public Health,* 12 (suppl.): S1–3.

You, J. and Wong, W. C. W. 2005. "The cost-effectiveness of an outreach clinical model in the management and prevention of gonorrhea and chlamydia among Chinese female sex workers in Hong Kong 2005". *Sexually Transmitted Diseases* (in press).

Appendix

List of some non-governmental organisations

All Round Service

Organisation	Address	Phone	Fax	Email
Yan Oi Tong	18 Kai Man Path, Tuen Mun, N.T.	26557788	26557799	yot@yanoitong.org.hk
Tung Wah Group of Hospitals	12 Po Yan Street, Sheung Wan, Hong Kong	28597500	28597859	enquiry@tungwah.org.hk
Po Leung Kuk	66 Leighton Road, Causeway Bay, Hong Kong	22778888	25764509	plkinfo@poleungkuk.org.hk
Chinese YMCA of Hong Kong	23 Waterloo Road, Kowloon, Hong Kong	27719111	27714096	info@ymca.org.hk
Caritas-Hong Kong	Room 602, Caritas House, 2 Caine Road, Hong Kong	25242071	25369213	info@caritas.org.hk
The Neighbourhood Advice-Action Council	Room 704, Duke of Windsor Social Service Building, 15 Hennessy Road, Wanchai, Hong Kong	25278888	25286552	ho@naac.org.hk

Patients

Organisation	Address	Phone	Fax	Email
Regeneration Society	G/F, 8–11,Yat Tung House, Tung Tau Estate, Kowloon	23826963	25637041	info@regensoc.org.hk
Alliance for Patients' Mutual Help Organizations	G/F, Wang Lai House, Wang Tau Hom Estate, Kowloon	23046371	30065999	main@apmho.org
The Hong Kong Society for Rehabilitation	6/F, 7 Sha Wan Drive, Pokfulam, Hong Kong	28176277	28551947	enquiry@rehabsociety.org.hk

Mental Handicap

Organisation	Address	Phone	Fax	Email
Hong Chi Association	Pinehill Village, Chung Nga Road, Nam Hang, Tai Po, N.T.	26891105	26614620	hdoffice@hongchi.org.hk

Organisation	Address	Phone	Fax	Email
Society for the Welfare of the Autistic Persons	Room 210–214, Block 19, Shek Kip Mei Estate, Kowloon	27883326	27781414	info@swap.org.hk
Fu Hong Society	G/F, 2A Po On Road, Cronin Garden, Sham Shui Po, Kowloon	27450424	27864097	fhs@fuhong.org
The Hong Kong Down Syndrome Association	G/F, 103–106, Wing Shui House, Lek Yuen Estate, Shatin, N.T.	26975391	26924955	hkdsa@hk-dsa.org.hk
The Society for the Relief of Disabled Children	The Duchess of Kent Children's Hospital at Sandy Bay, No. 12, Sandy Bay Road, Pokfulam, Hong Kong	28193050	28170322	info@srdc.org.hk
The Spastics Association of Hong Kong	Room 603, Duke of Windsor Social Service Building, 15 Hennessy Road, Wanchai, Hong Kong	25278978	28663727	ho@spastic.org.hk

Drug Abusers

Organisation	Address	Phone	Fax	Email
The Society for the Aid and Rehabilitation of Drug Abusers	3/F, Duke of Windsor Social Service Building, 15 Hennessy Road, Wanchai, Hong Kong	25277723	28652056	sarda@sarda.org.hk

Family Problems

Organisation	Address	Phone	Fax	Email
Mother's Choice	42B Kennedy Road, Mid-Levels, Hong Kong	25377633	25377681	admin@mothers choice.com
Against Child Abuse	107–108, G/F, Wai Yuen House, Chuk Yuen (North) Estate, Wong Tai Sin, Kowloon	23516060	27528483	webmaster@aca.org .hk
Harmony House	P.O. Box No. 99068, Tsim Sha Tsui Post Office, Kowloon	25220434	–	hhshelter@harmony househk.org
The Family Planning Association of Hong Kong	10/F, Southorn Centre, 130 Hennessy Road, Wanchai, Hong Kong	25754477	28346767	fpahk@famplan.org .hk

Organisation	Address	Phone	Fax	Email
Hong Kong Single Parents Association	No.1–7, G/F, Tung Moon House, Tai Hang Tung Estate, Shek Kip Mei, Kowloon	23381303	23375764	info@hkspa.org.hk

Elderly

Organisation	Address	Phone	Fax	Email
Helping Hand	1st Floor, 12 Borrett Road, Hong Kong	25224494	28401278	admin@helpinghand.org.hk
Hong Kong Alzheimer's Disease Association	G/F, Wang Yip House, Wang Tau Hom Estate, Kowloon	23381120	23380772	info@hkada.org.hk
Hong Kong Society for the Aged	7/F, Kai Seng Commercial Centre, 4–6 Hankow Road, Tsim Sha Tsui, Kowloon	25112235	25072417	info@sage.org.hk

Counselling

Organisation	Address	Phone	Fax	Email
Suicide Prevention Services	P.O. Box 83350, San Po Kong Post Office, Kowloon	23820000 23822007	23822004	admin@sps.org.hk
The Samaritan Befrienders Hong Kong	Unit 126–127, G/F, Kam Wah House, Choi Hung Estate, Kowloon	27908844	23436359	sbhkinfo@sbhk.org.hk

Children

Organisation	Address	Phone	Fax	Email
Children's Cancer Foundation	Room 702, Tung Ning Building,125 Connaught Road Central, Hong Kong	28152525	28155511	ccf@ccf.org.hk
Playright Children's Play Association	Flat A, 18/F, Block F, 3 Lok Man Road, Chai Wan, Hong Kong	28982922	28984539	info@playright.org.hk

Blind People

Organisation	Address	Phone	Fax	Email
Hong Kong Blind Union	Room 13–20, G/F, Tsui Ying House, Tsui Ping Estate, Kwun Tong, Kowloon	23390666	23387850	info@hkbu.org.hk

Organisation	Address	Phone	Fax	Email
The Hong Kong Society for the Blind	248 Nam Cheong Street, Sham Shui Po, Kowloon	27788332	27880040	enquiry@hksb.org.hk

Psychiatric Patients

Organisation	Address	Phone	Fax	Email
New Life Psychiatric Rehabilitation Association	332 Nam Cheong Street, Sham Shui Po, Kowloon	23324343	27709345	ho@nlpra.org.hk

Youth

Organisation	Address	Phone	Fax	Email
The Hong Kong Federation of Youth Groups	Room 1002, Duke of Windsor Social Service Building, 15 Hennessy Road, Wanchai, Hong Kong	25272448	25282105	hq@hkfyg.org.hk

Source: Homepage of The Hong Kong Council of Social Service (http://www.hkcss.org.hk/cm/mls/member/amliste2.asp).

SECTION II

Problem-based Diagnoses and
Management
in the General Population

Chapter 10

Tiredness

◆ Martin LINDSAY ◆

Scenario

A 45-year-old man comes to see you with a 4-week history of tiredness.

What are the likely diagnoses and how do you proceed to make a final diagnosis?

Causes generally can be divided into 3 groups:

1. The most likely
2. The important possibilities (i.e. must not forget even if unlikely)
3. The rare or unusual possibilities

The most likely causes

- Anaemia—due to poor diet or amenorrhoea
- Psychosocial
- Diabetes mellitus
- Hypothyroidism
- (Post-) Acute infection, e.g. infectious mononucleosis, influenza
- Alcohol abuse
- Drug abuse
- Excess use of caffeine-containing drinks or food affecting sleep patterns, e.g. coffee, chocolate, tea

The important possibilities that (may) need to be excluded

- Liver failure
- Renal failure
- Heart failure
- Malignancy including haematological
- Chronic infections, e.g. HIV, Hepatitis B or C, TB
- Other endocrine disorders, e.g. Cushing's, Addison's disease, hyperparathyroidism, hypopituitarism
- Iatrogenic, i.e. drugs such as β-blockers, antidepressants, anti-epileptics, cimetidine, antihistamines, antiemetics etc.

The rare or unusual possibilities

- Myasthenia gravis
- Multiple sclerosis
- Parkinson's disease
- Chronic obstructive pulmonary disease (COPD)
- Motor neurone disease
- Chronic fatigue syndrome
- Carbon monoxide poisoning
- Sleep apnoea
- Metabolic, e.g. hypokalaemia, hypomagnesaemia

Psychosocial

This is a particularly common presentation in the teens to 30s age group. Psychosocial covers a very broad range of possibilities from environmental factors (such as sleep depravation due to noise or jet lag), to post-stress reaction, e.g. after exams causing either elation or depression, to work or family problems, to anxiety-depression, and so on. Also be aware that if there is a mental health issue such as depression, there may be primary and secondary gain factors too.

Primary gain can be defined as a form of benefit due to the avoidance of an underlying predicament. Take this example: the patient may be too tired or exhausted to go to school/work so circumventing (at least temporarily) a particularly stressful situation. This could be because of, for example, an examination or a disciplinary procedure.

Secondary gain is where other tangible benefits occur from the avoidance behaviour (i.e. the primary gain), e.g. financial in the way of state benefits or permanently avoiding the underlying predicament of the primary gain.

Tertiary gain is about the carer gaining by replacing what the carer has now lost (usually self-worth by being previously deemed to be useful to family/society), e.g. looking after the currently "ill" patient after either having retired from work and having nothing else to occupy their time, or their children have left home having spent their whole married life looking after them.

Symptoms pattern

Just like dizziness, tiredness is a vague term. It is often described by the patient in many different ways: lethargy, no energy, listless, "feeling anyhow" and so forth.

Once this has been established, which usually takes seconds, the rest of the history is about trying to determine causation.

Specific questions to ask that may help

Given that in younger adults the problem is psychosocial in the majority of cases, it is worth asking the patient if they have any other symptoms apart from the tiredness. If they have not noticed anything it is often time-saving to head for the psychosocial issues. It is imperative, however, to tackle this with great sensitivity. Firstly, as the patient may feel by doing so you are belittling their symptoms or worse disbelieving them. Further, for some, it implies the doctor thinks they are "neurotic, it is all in the head and that the patient is wasting the doctor's time". Again it is essential to convey to the patient that any psychological problem is as important as any physical illness (which it is), that your time is not being wasted (which it is not) but that to assist the patient fully, the underlying cause should always be sought and if identified dealt with as this is the only sure way of achieving a cure.

Whilst a brief mental health assessment is vital, remember that the patient may not be depressed, just stressed. Thus, initially enquire about lifestyles, family or work problems and whether the patient feels they are stressed/under pressure. Also ask about their sleep patterns. If any of the foregoing gives a positive response, proceed to a full mental health assessment.

Always check for physical causes even if there seems to be a psychosocial cause. This is because occasionally a patient under psychosocial stress manages to cope until such time as they have one too many problems (in this case the physical illness). Their coping mechanisms then succumb. At that point in time they then have two broad problems: the physical (which may or may not be minor) and the psychosocial. If it transpires there is a definite case of mental health issues, the questions to be asked about physical causation can be brief. For example, consider any chest problems or shortness of breath (Is the weight and appetite normal?) rather than the full systematic approach.

Also remember that alcohol abuse or occasional drug abuse may be a reflection of an underlying psychological problem rather than the problem itself. For example, patients often use alcohol to alleviate insomnia due to anxieties or worries. Clearly excessive, prolonged alcohol use is serious and dangerous. However you may be seeing the patient before the addictive phase has been reached. Consequently by acknowledging their underlying problem, the doctor will not only treat the underlying problem but also prevent a secondary problem, namely addiction.

If there is/are no obvious psychosocial cause(s) then a more thorough physical enquiry will need to be made. As always remember the common aetiologies and concentrate on these before going onto the serious or rare possibilities. Always be wary of the elderly patient who has not visited a doctor for many years. Invariably there is something physically wrong. If these enquiries are also fruitless then you may need to rely on the investigations.

A 45-year-old man comes to see you with a 4-week history of tiredness and feeling exhausted all the time. He hardly ever comes to the surgery. He has a good relationship with his wife whom he has been married to for some 20 years and has 2 children aged 16 and 12. He is an accountant in a large company that is about to go onto the public stock exchange. Consequently, he is extremely busy at work. His sleep is therefore disturbed not only due to the pressure at work but also because his eldest child is about to take some important exams. In fact, he says, the whole household is feeling the pressure. His poor quality sleep, due to ruminations, presents both as initial insomnia and early morning wakening. Apart from the sleep issue, his appetite is normal but he is a bit overweight, no tearfulness, concentration is somewhat under par due to the tiredness but essentially all right. He denies depression or anxiety and he feels optimistic about the future.

Systematic enquiry reveals nothing of note. In particular no history of any viral-like illnesses. No polyuria, polydipsia.

He eats 3 times a day, though a bit erratically, but ensures he eats fruit and vegetables daily. He drinks no more than 4 cups of tea daily and no coffee. He is on no medication, smokes 20 cigarettes per day for over 20 years and drinks 8 units of alcohol per week. He denies illicit drug use.

A working diagnosis

Diabetes mellitus, hypothyroidism, alcohol abuse, drug abuse, diet and excess use of caffeine do not appear to be relevant on history.

Similarly, the "important possibilities" are not likely, given the history. However they have not been fully excluded. Note that he is a heavy smoker (pack years = 20). It is also noteworthy that he has never been seen before for stress-related problems. Indeed he hardly ever sees a doctor.

Having said all that and based on the history, a working diagnosis has to be an Acute Stress Reaction.

Examination

In all cases of tiredness, examination of the cardiovascular system, respiratory system and abdomen should take place.

Scenario

In this particular situation, it was noted that he was slightly jaundiced. He also had slight hepatomegaly (1–2 finger breadth, smooth, non-tender). No lymphadenopathy, splenomegaly, clubbing, anaemia, oedema or cyanosis. Examination of the cardiovascular and respiratory systems was normal.

Reviewing the history

Classically, a history is followed by the examination and then the investigation(s). In real life situations it is not uncommon to have to revisit the history in the light of clinical findings or test results.

The situation here has now changed. The patient had not noticed the jaundice, as it was only mild. Thus having made a finding, the clinician has to review the history.

Scenario

On pointing out his jaundice, the patient was surprised and also concerned. He had not noticed the problem. Nor had he any history suggestive of any viral-type illnesses. He was not in a high risk group of getting Hepatitis B/C or HIV.

Clinical diagnosis

The working diagnosis has now dramatically changed in the light of the examination findings. It includes all the possibilities of jaundice. The next step is the investigations.

Investigations

Blood tests

The following tests are used for routine purposes. Clearly, other investigations are possible and are dependent on the history obtained.

Full Blood Count	To exclude anaemia and other haematological possibilities
Erythrocyte Sedimentation Rate (ESR)	General screen including for connective tissue diseases
Urea and Electrolytes	Renal function and indicator of possible metabolic problem
Liver Function Tests	Liver function
Thyroid Function Tests	Thyroid disease
Glucose	To exclude diabetes mellitus
Monospot/Infectious Mononucleosis test	Glandular Fever
Gamma Gluteryl Transferase	Especially if alcohol abuse is suspected
C Reactive Protein	More sensitive test for infection, connective tissue disease or malignancy
Urinalysis	Another check for diabetes and nitrates or microalbuminium
Mid Stream Urine	To exclude covert urinary tract infection

Other general tests

These are very much dependent on history and could include the following (this list is not exhaustive):

Chest X-ray	Malignancy or TB especially if any respiratory or weight symptoms
HIV	If lifestyle (e.g. practising male homosexual, drug abuser or partner of either of the former categories) suggests and ONLY after the patient has been counselled. Also consider if from African continent or South-East Asia simply due to the prevalence in those areas

Hepatitis B or C	If possible liver pathology on history, examination or lifestyle suggests and ONLY after the patient has been counselled (see HIV above). If have been in contact with someone with this illness
Hepatitis A	If possible liver pathology on history or examination. If risk of contact from lifestyle, e.g. recently been to an endemic area

Given the examination findings, all the above tests would be performed. The exception would be HIV as there was nothing in his lifestyle to suggest it should be done at this point in time. However if the tests came back confirming a hepatitic picture (i.e. inflamed liver) and the hepatitis screens were all normal, then HIV would have to be reconsidered.

If, on the other hand, the liver function tests confirmed not a hepatitic but obstructive picture, then urgent upper abdominal ultrasound (liver, gallbladder, spleen and pancreas) would need to be arranged.

Findings and results

The blood results are all normal except that his gamma gluteryl transferase is twice the normal upper limit and his alanine transferase is marginally raised though his aspartame transaminase and alkaline phosphatase are normal.

Management of tiredness

Initial management

This clearly raises the possibility of some form of obstructive liver disease. The following tests would therefore be reasonable to conduct:

- Ultrasound scan of upper abdomen, i.e. liver, gall bladder, pancreas and spleen
- Autoantibodies especially smooth muscle and mitochondrial (for auto-immune hepatitis)
- Immunoglobulins (for auto-immune hepatitis)
- Ceruloplasmin/Copper levels (Wilson's disease—rare)

- Coagulation studies (if has liver disease and wish to ensure normal liver function)
- Ferritin (to exclude haemosiderosis)
- Alpha-1 antitripsin (cystic fibrosis—extremely rare in Hong Kong)
- Alpha feto-protein (tumour marker)

Findings and results

All the new blood tests were normal. The scan showed fatty liver change but all the other organs were normal.

Follow-up management

The results were explained to the patient. The most likely cause of the liver problem was non-alcoholic fatty liver disease (NAFLD) and was not related to his tiredness, which is due to the stress at home and in his work.

The NAFLD is thought to be due to insulin resistance and heralds the possible onset of diabetes. The management is initially lifestyle changes. Reduce weight and increase exercise. Keep alcohol intake to below recommended levels (21 units per week for men and 14 units per week for women).

Monitoring is important as some 3–4% of patients can progress to cirrhosis (Matteoni et al. 1999). There may be an indication to use insulin sensitising drugs such as metformin or the newer thazolidinediones, e.g. rosiglitazone and/or lipid lowering drugs such as the fibrates. Statins have no role in NAFLD. The use of these drugs is very much under the auspices of a hepatologist.

A rare variant is non-alcoholic steatohepatitis (NASH). This is very important as 25% can progress to cirrhosis and 11% can die from it (Matteoni et al. 1999). Liver biopsy may be indicated, as this is the only sure way of confirming the diagnosis. Thus referral to a hepatologist may well be indicated.

In this particular instance the patient was advised about lifestyle changes and his liver function tests (LFT) were reviewed three months later. By that time he had lost weight and was exercising regularly. His LFT were improving. His daughter had passed her examinations. He had delegated some of his work and as a consequence of all the changes he felt better.

Summary

Not all physical ailments can cause tiredness. Some can be totally incidental. Some could herald future possible problems.

In this case whilst the presentation was tiredness and due to psycho-social problems, there was a physical disease. The identification of this disease led to alteration of lifestyle which, hopefully would defer or possibly prevent future illnesses.

Similarly the acknowledgement of the psychosocial issues also led to changes in both work practices and also contributed to the patient's decision to increase exercise. This too would help to prevent/defer not only physical illness but also mental well-being.

Reference

Matteoni et al. 1999. "Non-alcoholic fatty liver disease: A spectrum of clinical and pathological severity". *Gastroenterology*, 116: 1413–1419.

Chapter 11

Shortness of Breath

◆ Martin LINDSAY ◆

Scenario

Mr. W is a 55-year-old office worker. He has been smoking 20 cigarettes a day for some 35 years. For the last few months he has been having a persistent cough. Initially he thought it was a "smokers' cough" but is now not so sure as he is also getting some occasional wheezing and shortness of breath. He is on no medication and rarely sees his family doctor.

What are the likely diagnoses and how do you proceed to make a final diagnosis?

The most likely causes

- Asthma
- Chronic obstructive pulmonary diseases (COPD)

The important possibilities that (may) need to be excluded

- Cancer
- Infection, e.g. tuberculosis
- Pulmonary emboli (PE)
- Cardiac

The rare or unusual possibilities

- Sarcoid

- Interstitial lung disease, e.g. cryptogenic fibrosing alveolitis (CFA)
- ENT pathology, e.g. post nasal drip or vocal cord dysfunction
- Bronchiectasis
- Gastro-intestinal reflux

Symptoms are not unique

The trouble with respiratory symptoms is that many diseases have similar symptoms. You can get wheezing, shortness of breath or cough in COPD, asthma, bronchiectasis, cardiac causes, infections, sarcoid, interstitial lung disease and so forth. Thus it is often the pattern of those symptoms or the presence of other symptoms that may help to differentiate.

For example, if the patient has green phlegm, it indicates infection and conditions such as asthma, COPD or bronchiectasis are prone to infection. As a generality, if it occurs only occasionally it is more likely asthma. If copious and daily then bronchiectasis is more likely. COPD is somewhere in between as they tend to have a degree of phlegm (though not usually green).

Symptoms pattern

By this one means the frequency, duration, precipitating and relieving factors, and whether the symptoms occur at any particular time of the day.

Wheezing

By definition asthma involves chronically inflamed, hyper-responsive airways. The generalised but variable airway obstruction is reversible either spontaneously or with the use of drugs. Thus it would be reasonable to expect an asthmatic to be asymptomatic most of the time but to have wheezing of variable severity at other times and due to hyper-responsiveness to have triggers that make symptoms worse (as in this case).

In contrast, COPD is a chronic, slowly progressive disorder characterised by airways obstruction that does not change markedly over several months (except in exacerbation when it suddenly gets worse). The impairment of lung function is largely fixed but is partially reversible by drugs. Thus the symptoms should be present all the time with possible exacerbations. Again this is more or less what occurs.

Specific questions to ask that may help

- It is therefore essential to ask Mr. W not only whether he coughs, wheezes and has shortness of breath but also when, how often and what makes the symptoms better or worse

- It would also be essential to ask if he has phlegm. If yes, what is the colour, consistency, volume and frequency. Using the same principle as above, if clear and frothy it would imply cardiac failure, if bloody, tumours or PE for example

- Does he have a history of atopy or as a child a history of recurrent coughs or wheezing? He may not have been told he had asthma as a child

- Is there a family history of atopy?

- Does aspirin or non-steroidal anti-inflammatory drugs (NSAIDs) make him wheeze? (10% of asthmatics cannot take aspirin or NSAIDs for this reason)

- Any chest pain? (PE, angina)

- Any weight loss? (tumours, TB)

- Always ask the patient what their concerns may be— you cannot reassure anyone until you know for certain what is bothering them

Pack years

You may come across this term. It is a useful way of standardising and therefore comparing the amount an individual has smoked. If less than 10 pack years, the probability of them having COPD is unlikely (unless they have other predisposing factors). To calculate:

$$\text{total pack years} = \frac{\text{number of cigarettes smoked per day}}{20^*} \times \text{number of years smoked}$$

(* = average number of cigarettes per pack)

So, for Mr. W: $20 \div 20 \times 35 = 35$ pack years

A working diagnosis

By the time you are about to examine the patient, you should have tried to establish if your original list of likely, serious, not to forget and unusual diagnoses are still the same. In other words have you formed a working diagnosis?

The examination is then to help confirm or refute the working diagnoses.

Examination

General

Oedema (heart failure), cyanosis (severity of shortness of breath), clubbing (CFA, bronchiectasis, tumours), lymphadenopathy (TB, tumours), or anaemia (is this the aetiology of his shortness of breath).

Cardiovascular

Blood pressure, pulse, apex beat, jugular venous pressure heart sounds (for cardiac causes).

Respiratory

Examination is usually normal in asthma except during exacerbations when bilateral expiratory wheezing should be heard. If unilateral, an alternative diagnosis should be considered such as pneumonia, tumours, inhaled foreign body etc.

Fine basal crepitations (cryptogenic fibrosing alveolitis) med-coarse crepitations (heart failure, chest infections etc.), evidence of other lung pathology, e.g. pleural effusions (heart failure, tumours, infections).

Peak expiratory flow rate (PEFR)—see below under "Other investigations—Lung function tests".

Some authorities, including the authors, feel that PEFR are so intrinsic to the examination of the respiratory system that unless performed one cannot say that a full respiratory examination has been done. However it has been placed below as technically it is an investigation.

Clinical diagnosis

After the examination a clinical diagnosis should have been reached. It may still consist of several different possibilities but some possibilities should have been excluded by now. For example, no phlegm on history, no oedema, no tachycardia and no crepitations then heart failure is not a likely problem.

Investigations

 Remember, investigations are both time consuming (for the patient and others, e.g. radiologists, radiographers etc.) and cost money. Thus they should only be done to assist in making or excluding a potential diagnosis. They certainly should not be done on a blanket basis. Occasionally there may be extenuating circumstances, e.g. medico-legal, or a disabled person who has great difficulty in getting to a hospital. However these are the notable exceptions.

Blood tests

- Complete blood count (looking for anaemia or secondary polycythaemia)
- ESR (useful screen—if raised consider TB, tumours, sarcoid, interstitial lung disease)
- C-reactive protein (indicating TB, other infections or tumours)
- Serum angiotensin converting enzyme (only if sarcoid is a good possibility)
- Calcium levels (only if sarcoid or tumours are a possibility)
- D-dimer (useful screen for excluding low or medium risk of PE)
- Liver function tests (again if tumours a possibility)
- Thyroid function test—hypothyroidism can cause muscle weakness and so cause shortness of breath. Hyperthyroidism can lead to cardiac failure. Thyroid disease is the only endocrine cause of shortness of breath
- Urea and electrolytes (only if heart failure on history or examination)

Other investigations

- Plain chest X-ray. This is essential for any new "wheezer". It helps to exclude both heart failure and other lung pathologies. It does NOT confirm either asthma or COPD. Hyper-inflated lungs can be seen in either condition but both diagnoses are clinically-based and in the case of COPD need spirometry too

- Lung function tests. These can be divided into two types: peak flow meters and spirometry proper

Peak flow meters are helpful due to their size, ease of use and cheapness. They are useful too in any one individual in that any change can be easily seen. All family doctor clinics should have them. However they are not as accurate as spirometers, nor are their results as reproducible.

The commonest way of using a peak flow meter is the diurnal chart: the best of three blows is noted and charted. It is performed immediately upon waking and again around 4–6 p.m. over a 2-week period. The blows must be before any inhaler is used. A non-asthmatic has an 8% variation in their PEFR. A variation of 15% is suggestive of asthma. A 20% swing confirmatory (provided history and examination are compatible with the diagnosis of asthma).

An alternative method used for the occasional asthmatic is for them to determine their normal baseline PEFR and to then check their peak flow whenever they are symptomatic.

Other methods employed to ascertain variability is to check a baseline peak flow chart and to repeat the chart either after a 2-week course of 30mg prednisolone daily or after 8–12 weeks on a high dose inhaled corticosteroid, e.g. beclometasone 1000 mcg twice a day. Some would also check PEFR after exercise or after giving a short acting β_2-agonist.

Spirometry is essential to confirm the diagnosis of COPD and at times asthma too. The minimum parameters to be measured are vital capacity (VC), forced vital capacity (FVC) and forced expiratory volume (FEV1). In COPD the VC may be greater than FVC (due to airway collapsing because of reduced lung architecture with the forced expiration). The FEV1 is reduced and does not return to normal with either steroids or bronchodilators. Ideally loop-flow charts are also helpful to establish if there is restrictive as opposed to obstructive pattern.

Other lung function tests, e.g. gas transfer are helpful to determine if there is any lung (as opposed to airway) pathology. However these are purely hospital-based type of investigations.

Findings and results

The rest of the history and examination was unremarkable other than a PEFR reading that was below the normal range for his age, gender, ethnicity and height.

This therefore leaves asthma or COPD as the real possibilities. It would be reasonable to conclude that cardiac, ENT and gastroenterology pathologies have reasonably been excluded, but not the other lung pathologies at this time.

Why only reasonably? Sometimes if a patient is not responding to treatment, a doctor has to review all the original possibilities again.

Management of shortness of breath

Initial management

This is going to assume that as the family doctor, you do not have access to spirometry.

- Arrange blood tests and chest X-ray (see above)
- Start salbutamol (the patient needs symptomatic relief)
- Start diurnal peak flow chart
- Review 2 weeks later

Note 1: If you, as the family doctor, have access to spirometry then you will still perform the above but also perform spirometry at this stage.

Note 2: Inhaled corticosteroids should NOT be started at this time until infective possibilities have first been excluded.

Two-week follow-up management

If the blood tests and chest X-ray are unremarkable, thus either asthma or COPD is likely to be the diagnosis.

The patient finds a trial of salbutamol helpful. This neither confirms nor refutes either asthma or COPD as improvement can occur in either condition.

However if his peak flow chart shows no diurnal variation and is still low, this would strongly indicate COPD. Asthma is still a possibility—does he have significant reversibility? Thus either way you can now safely proceed to a trial of steroid as infections and other serious pathologies have been excluded.

NOTE: If there was a diurnal variation it could be adult onset asthma or COPD with a significant degree of reversibility (also known as mixed asthma/COPD).

Trial of steroids

A 2-week course of oral prednisolone or inhaled beclometasone (or equivalent) 1000 mcg twice a day is given for 6 weeks (minimum) to 3 months. Provided there are no medical contra-indications for the oral route, both oral or inhaled methods are acceptable and so the decision can lie with the patient (British Thoracic Society 2006). A pressurised meter dose inhaler via a spacer device ensures adequate intake and reduces local (oral) side-effects of the inhaled beclometasone.

Scenario

Mr. W is told to continue with his peak flow chart and to return at the end of the steroid trial period.

Post-steroid trial review

Interpretation of results

There are three possible results:

1. Complete reversibility: in which case the diagnosis is adult onset asthma
2. No change to the peak flow readings: this would then confirm COPD
3. Partial Reversibility, i.e. the peak flows are better but still not in the normal range. This lends to the diagnosis of COPD with partial reversibility (mixed asthma/COPD)

Mr. W's chart showed partial reversibility.

If spirometry is available then a trial of steroids would need to be performed if the initial results show an obstructive picture. The various outcomes are identical, i.e.

- Complete reversibility, i.e. the FEVl in 1 second is greater than 400 ml or the FEV1 returns to normal. In which case the diagnosis is adult onset asthma

- No change to the peak flow readings, i.e. the FEV1 increase is less than 200 ml—this would then confirm COPD

- Partial reversibility, i.e. the FEV1 is between 201 and 399 ml. This lends to the diagnosis of COPD with partial reversibility (mixed asthma/COPD)

Drug management of COPD

- Use pressurised multi-dose inhalers (pMDI) with a spacer device.

  This is by far the most cost effective method. There has been no evidence that breath actuated inhalers are in any way superior except for those who cannot use or tolerate pMDIs

- Check inhaler technique and compliance at any stage if patient is still symptomatic

- Short acting β_2-agonist (SABA), e.g. salbutamol, on an as needed basis

- Add short acting anticholinergic (SAA), e.g. ipratropium, if still symptomatic, also on an as needed basis

- Add regular use of a long acting β_2-agonist (LABA), e.g. salmeterol or formoterol to SABA and SAA

- Add regular use of a long acting anticholinergic, e.g. tiotropium, to LABA and SABA and SAA

  Tiotropium is a promising relatively new drug. There is some evidence to suggest it is superior to salmeterol but there have been limited number of studies thus far. So at this time it is best to add in after a LABA.

- ICS should be started in all patients who show a positive response to a steroid trial or those with moderate/severe COPD who have 2 or more exacerbations per year IRRESPECTIVE of steps 1 to 4 above
- Add a xanthene if patient still symptomatic despite the seven points above
- Influenza vaccination annually for all
- Consider nebuliser therapy
- Consider oxygen therapy (both long-term and ambulatory)
- Consider referral to a respiratory physician

More advanced management of COPD

By the end of the above a final diagnosis should have been reached. However the family doctor may not have access to spirometry. So how can a diagnosis of COPD be made?

Two other possibilities

1. Increased forced expiratory time

   To determine forced expiratory time:

   The individual takes as deep a breath as possible. The person then opens the mouth wide and exhales as fast as possible. The exhalation time is then measured in seconds.

   Normal is 2–5 seconds.

   A value of 6 seconds suggests, and greater than 9 seconds probably indicates, COPD.

2. Care study (Straus 2000)

   If: 1. > 40 pack years AND 2. > 45 years old AND 3. Maximum laryngeal height < 4 cm.

   The probability of having COPD is 96%.

   If none of the above is present, the probability is < 1%.

   Adding history of COPD has minimal effect at altering the % risk.

   Laryngeal height (distance between the top of the thyroid cartilage and the suprasternal notch): At end-expiration with the patient sitting up, looking straight ahead and with hands relaxed in their lap, palpate the top of the thyroid cartilage which is readily identified by the notch on its superior edge. Hook your index finger over the thyroid cartilage and using the rest of your fingers, measure the distance from the top of the thyroid cartilage to the sternal notch in finger-breadths. Convert these finger-breadths to centimetres and record this distance.

References

"British guideline on the management of asthma. Section 2: Diagnosis & natural history". Retrieved 17 January, 2006, from http://www.sign.ac.uk/guidelines/fulltext/63/section2.html.

Straus, S. E., McAlister, F. A., Sackett, D. L. and Deeks, J. J. 2000. "The accuracy of patient history, wheezing, and laryngeal measurements in diagnosing obstructive airway disease". *Journal of American Medical Association*, 283: 1853–1857.

Chapter 12

Chest Pain

◆ YIU Yuk Kwan ◆

Scenario

Mr. Wong, a 47-year-old postman, complained of chest discomfort for about 2 months. His wife accompanied him during the visit. He used to be a fit trail walker but has seldom exercised in the recent few months. He attributed this to tiredness with the increasing workload.

He experienced on-and-off vague lower retrosternal discomfort which was poorly defined and was sometimes associated with lifting heavy objects. The pain would only last a few minutes provided he would rest and rub the affected area. He could then continue to work. He was not very concerned about this pain but last night he experienced another similar attack which had been witnessed by his wife. He comes to your surgery today, accompanied by his wife, just wanting to get your reassurance in order to keep his wife happy.

What are the likely diagnoses and how do you proceed to make a final diagnosis?

The most likely causes

- Local trauma
- Referral pain from spine
- Ischaemic heart disease
- Oesophageal (spasm or oesophagitis)

- Costochondritis/Musculo-skeletal
- Paroxysmal anxiety disorder (panic attacks)

The important possibilities that (may) need to be excluded

- Acute myocardial infarction
- Pneumonia/Infected pleurisy
- Lung tumour causing erosion or pleurisy
- Acute pulmonary embolism
- Upper gastro-intestinal ulcers
- Aortic dissection
- Sub-phrenic abscess

The rare or unusual possibilities

- Other psychogenic aetiologies–somatisation
- Shingles
- Cholecystitics
- Pericarditis
- Pneumothorax
- Chronic pulmonary embolism, i.e. multiple minor pulmonary embolism can cause minor episodes of shortness of breath with or without minor episodes of chest pain, and thus can be a hard diagnosis to make

Differential diagnoses of chest pain

Cardiac causes

- Angina pectoris
- Unstable angina
- Myocardial infarction
- Pericarditis, aortic dissection (rarer cause)

Non-cardiac causes

- Pulmonary causes—pulmonary embolism, pneumothorax, cancer, pleural disease
- Neuromuscular causes—chest wall pain due to costochrondritis

(Tietze's syndrome), herpes zoster preceding the development of the vesicular rash eruption and persisting after the rash subsided

- Gastrointestinal causes—reflux oesophagitis, oesophageal spasm, peptic ulcer disease gastritis, cholecystitis, sub-phrenic abscess
- Psychological causes—panic attack and depression
- Referred pain from spine
- Local trauma

Differences in presentation (Table 12.1)

Clinical features suggesting anginal pain

Anginal pain is often described as a squeezing, heaviness or pressure sensation lasting 2–20 minutes. Classically it is aggravated by exertion, emotional stress or eating.

Clinical features suggesting non-anginal pain

- Pain that is sharp stabbing in nature, aggravated by inspiration, very brief/long lasting, i.e. for seconds, or lasting for days or weeks
- Pain that is localised within the span of one finger
- Pain that can be reproduced by movement or palpation of chest wall or arms
- Repetition

 Risk factors that increase the likelihood of angina include prior history of myocardial infarction (history or ECG), age > 65 (risk increases with age), 2 anginal events in last 24 hours, aspirin within the last 7 days, history of diabetes mellitus/hyperlipidaemia, being a smoker, history of hypertension, positive family history of ischaemic heart disease, obesity or ST-segment changes in ECG.

In some studies, risk scores are given to the above with 1 point for each risk factor. A risk score of < 4 with pain subsided is considered as low risk of acute coronary syndrome (Ebell 2001; Sabatine et al. 2002; Morrow et al. 2000).

Table 12.1 The difference between classical anginal and non-anginal pain

	Anginal	Non-anginal
Nature of pain	Squeezing, heaviness, pressing discomfort	Sharp, stabbing*
Site	Poorly localised in retrosternal area, anterior chest, epigastrium	Localised especially neuromuscular causes (can be poorly localised for psychogenic causes)
Radiation	Typically radiates to left arm, neck or jaw	Depending on aetiology (thoracic outlet syndrome can radiate from chest to upper arm)
Duration	2–20 minutes (for unstable angina, can be > 20 minutes)	Seconds or days or weeks
Aggravating factor	Exertion (resting for unstable angina) Emotional stress Eating (usually a very large meal) Cold weather = Condition that increases myocardial oxygen demand	Vigorous or unaccustomed exertion (muscular or ligamentous strain) Inspiration for pleuritis
Relieving factor	Rest (except unstable angina) and relief within minutes Sublingual GTN: usually relief within 5 minutes	Note: GTN can also relieve pain due to oesophageal spasm
Associated features	Diaphoresis, dyspnoea, nausea or vomiting	
Red flag sign		Tachypnoea, dyspnoea and hypoxemia—consider pulmonary embolisation (see history of risk factors below)

* Sharp and stabbing pains do not completely exclude ischaemic cause. 22% of patients with ischaemic heart disease diagnosed in Accident & Emergency Department were complaining of sharp pain (American College of Emergency Physicians 1995).

Pulmonary embolism risk factors

1. Past history of a thrombo-embolic event

2. Recent immobilisation, e.g. long haul flight (> 8 hours); recent operation; leg in a plaster cast

3. Patient taking a pro-thrombotic medication, e.g. combined oral contraceptive, tamoxifen

4. Known pro-thrombotic genetic disorder, e.g. Factor V Leiden

5. Family history of thrombo-embolism in a patient that has not been screened for risk of pro-thrombo-embolism

6. Medical disorders that promote risk of thrombo-embolism, e.g. sickle cell disease

Diagnosing pulmonary embolism

This is notoriously difficult. The classical trilogy of acute onset chest pain, shortness of breath and haemoptysis are not often present. D-Dimer is good at excluding pulmonary emboli in low and medium risk groups but not among the high risk ones. ECG or chest x-ray changes are invariably not present. This therefore leaves only ventilation/perfusion (V/Q) and CTPA (Computer Tomography Pulmonary Artery) perfusion scans as the definitive procedures (different doctors have different views as to the superiority of one over the other). Certainly if there is abnormality to the pulmonary architecture then CTPA is preferable, whereas in a person with normal pulmonary architecture V/Q scans are cheaper, require far less radiation and invariably are just as adequate. However in primary care neither is available and the best way to diagnose suspected pulmonary embolism is to consider it in all cases of chest pain/shortness of breath.

Physical examination

Physical examination should be focused based on the working diagnosis generated. Seek relevant and discriminating physical signs to help you confirm or refute the working diagnosis. In patients with acute pain, if the history is highly suggestive of a serious cardiovascular cause, the patient should be referred to hospital immediately.

General examination and vital signs such as tachypnoea, tachycardia and poor perfusion in a patient with acute chest pain are highly suggestive of serious cardiac causes. If cardiac causes are highly suspected, examination should be focused on delineating evidence of other complications from atherosclerotic disease like peripheral vascular disease, cerebrovascular disease and congestive heart failure. The general physical examination of patients with ischaemic heart disease is usually normal but:

- Xanthoma, xanthelasma and arcus senilis in a patient under 50 years of age are suggestive of hypercholesterolemia
- Vital signs like respiratory rate should be noted if patient is tachypnoeic
- Pulse rate should be noted to delineate tachycardia
- Blood pressure should be checked to denote any hypertension, which is one cardiovascular risk factor. Hypotension, on the other hand, is a poor prognostic sign for acute coronary heart syndrome. Asymmetry of blood pressure in the arm with asymmetrical pulse is suggestive of thoracic aortic dissection
- Jugular venous pressure should be determined to note any elevation suggestive of heart failure or inferior vena cava syndrome
- Peripheral pulses should be examined to delineate peripheral artery bruits as well as asymmetry especially of arm pulse, which is diagnostic of thoracic aortic dissection
- Arterial Blood Pressure Index (comparing blood pressure in the arm at the ante-cubital fossa with the blood pressure in the foot pulses) to delineate if there is any peripheral vascular disease in patients presenting with a history suggestive of peripheral vascular disease
- Fundi to observe retinal arteriolar changes
- Examination of the heart includes localising the apex beat. Significant displacement of the apex beat to the left indicates cardiac enlargement as in heart failure and left ventricular hypertrophy. Quality of cardiac impulse should also be noted. Forceful and sustained impulse is suggestive of left ventricular hypertrophy due to long standing hypertension, aortic stenosis or hypertrophic cardiomyopathy
- Heart sound to denote any soft first heart sound (S1) and paradoxically split second heart sound (S2) which reflect significant left ventricular dysfunction. Cardiac gallop which means an audible third heart sound (S3) also implies severe left ventricular failure or significant atrial regurgitation or mitural regurgitation. Presence of S3 and

development of fourth heart sound (S4) may be transient and occurring only during chest pain

A new apical systolic murmur can be found in some patients with ischaemia or infarction due to papillary muscle dysfunction and secondary mitral regurgitation or ventricular septal defect. This murmur may sometimes be present only during episodes of chest pain and strongly suggests myocardial ischaemia as a cause of the chest pain. Hence, during symptomatic episode, the findings of a new mitral regurgitation murmur, S3 or S4 gallop, or precordial lift, all suggest a high likelihood of coronary artery disease.

- Precordial rub should be checked in patients suspected of pleuritis or pericarditis. They are best detected with the diaphragm of the stethoscope. Pleural rub is heard during the inspiratory phase of respiration whilst pericardial rub can be heard throughout the respiratory cycle.

- Accentuated pulmonic component of the second heart sound and a new tricuspid regurgitant murmur is diagnostic of acute pulmonary hypertension from severe pulmonary embolisation

On the other hand, if the chest pain is of non-cardiac origin, physical examination should focus on other areas:

- An anxious, sighing, hyperventilating individual is more likely to be suffering from an anxiety disorder. However considering the whole clinical picture including detailed psychosocial assessment is very important since emotional stress can also precipitate anginal attack. Patients with anginal pain and in distress can also be anxious

- Patient should be inspected for signs of trauma and the rash of herpes zoster

- Chest pain of musculoskeletal origin is reproduced by palpation of chest wall or certain passive movements such as abduction, adduction or extension of the arms. There may be some "trigger points" on the chest wall

- Pneumothorax may be diagnosed by unilateral decreased breath sound and increased resonance. However a small pneumothorax (say 10 to 20% collapse) is unlikely to produce significant physical signs. Thus chest x-ray is the only way of making the diagnosis. In tension pneumothorax, trachea deviation may be detected

- Abdominal examination may be normal in patients with oesophageal spasm and reflux or peptic ulcer disease. Right upper quadrant tenderness or epigastric tenderness with deep inspiration may be detected in patients with cholecystitis (Murphy's sign)

Questions that may arise from the diagnosis

The key to diagnosis of chest pain remains in the medical history. Important questions to ask include the ones listed in Table 12.1: nature of the pain, its location, duration, intensity and radiation, aggravating or relieving factors, relationship with exertion, associated symptoms.

Investigations

Estimate the probability of ischaemic heart disease based on history first. This can be inferred using the estimates made by Diamond and Forrester (1979):

1. High probability situations (> 75%): men > 40 and women > 50 with typical anginal pain
2. Moderate probability (> 50%): men > 40 and women > 60 with atypical features or men < 40 and women < 50 with typical anginal pain
3. Low probability (< 20%): men < 40 and women < 50 with atypical features

Each patient must be evaluated INDIVIDUALLY and no single test provides 100% diagnostic accuracy. Then based on the pre-test probability select an appropriate strategy for subsequent tests:

1. If low probability of serious cardiac causes, investigation may not be necessary. Possible investigations that may be included are baseline blood test to assess the cardiovascular risk such as lipid profile, especially in a case with other cardiovascular risk factors, e.g. smoker. Chest x-ray may be needed to rule out other pulmonary causes. Resting ECG does not help to rule out chronic ischaemic changes but may be needed for reassurance of an anxious patient who is symptomatic. This should not be used unless there is a strong patient need for some "objective" reassurance and patient should be warned that a positive result is most likely to be a false positive result.

2. For moderate probability, an exercise ECG is the most useful test. The decision to use radionuclide scan depends on a balance between the benefit of additional information and the possible cost incurred.

    Exercise ECG is relatively inexpensive and provides sensitivity and specificity of 0.68 and 0.77 respectively (Garber and Soloman 1999). Incremental treadmill speed and elevation until the maximal heart rate for age is achieved. The patient is monitored for symptoms like chest pain, ECG changes, blood pressure as well as ventricular arrythmias. Interpretation is difficult for cases where maximal heart rate cannot be achieved.

    Exercise testing is not indicated for those who are unable to exercise because of claudication, spinal stenosis, arthritis, other causes of gait or instability, frailty, or with underlying ECG abnormalities that make standard ECG changes unreadable. For example pre-exisiting LVH with strain and left bundle branch block. Other contraindications to stress testing include unstable angina, severe aortic stenosis, unstable arrythmias and recent myocardial infarction (4–6 weeks).

    Other modalities of stress testing are available for patients who are unable to exercise, which also have higher sensitivity and specificity (please refer to "Advanced management" below).

3. High pre-test probability of stable anginal presentation. The investigation is aimed mainly at estimating the prognosis and stratifying the risk, principally to determine the amount of myocardium at risk. Resting ECG needed to detect any prior silent myocardial infarction. Post-infarction angina is a sign of potentially severe coronary heart disease. Radionuclide or echocardiographic stress testing can help to delineate the extent of myocardium at risk as well as segmental wall akinesis.

    If high pre-test probability of myocardial infarction or unstable angina is suspected, patients need to be sent to the emergency unit of a hospital without delay. For those with ECG changes on arrival in the emergency room, immediate angiography without prior non-invasive testing is a more cost-effective diagnostic approach.

    In such cases, especially when patients are in acute pain, resting ECG is a useful initial diagnostic test. The diagnosis can be based on ST-T wave morphology during symptomatic phase. ST segment elevation ≥ 1 mm in 2 or more consecutive leads is highly suggestive of acute myocardial infarction (MI) and associated with highest mortality and morbidity. ST segment depression of ≥ 1 mm or T wave inversion in two or more contiguous leads also strongly suggests ischaemia or acute MI. Presence of Q waves ≥ 0.04 seconds indicates previous MI. ECG abnormalities are strong positive predicators but as many as 82% of patients with acute coronary syndromes related chest pain have normal or near normal ECGs (Fesmire et al. 1998). As patients may have normal ECG initially, serial ECGs are needed to observe the evolution. However just routine use of resting ECG is not diagnostic of coronary heart disease since there are high false positives, especially for ST depression.

For cases with specific changes of ST or T-wave changes indicative of ischaemia, prompt consideration of therapy like thrombolytic or re-vascularisation should be given. Coronary angiogram is more cost effective than stress testing.

Advanced management

For patients with intermediate pre-test probability of angina

Exercise ECG with thallium or technetium sestamibi or single photon emission computed tomography (SPECT), which enhances sensitivity and specificity as well as three-dimensional views. It can be performed by treadmill exercising or adenosine or dipyridamole injection. The latter are coronary vasodilators and are used when patients are unable to exercise. Areas of redistribution suggests ischaemia whilst persistent defects suggest infarction.

Stress echocardiography can be performed by bicycle exercise or dobutamine stimulation. It detects wall motion abnormality. Cost is somewhat higher than resting ECG but sensitivity and specificity are better. The disadvantages include difficulty in imaging for obese patients and the need to image as close to peak exercise rate as possible. Dobutamine echocardiogram can be a method of choice for patients unable to exercise. Echo stress tests proved to be one of the most cost effective diagnostic tests in persons with an intermediate pre-test probability of coronary disease (Kuntz et al. 1999).

Positron emission tomography (PET) is the most sensitive and specific test for coronary insufficiency (Garber and Solomon 1999). However with its high cost and limited availability, it should be limited to selected cases.

Coronary angiogram: Because of the inherent risks and high costs, coronary angiography is reserved for cases with high probability of MI, unstable angina or those with persistent symptoms despite medical therapy. As diagnosis is closely tied to therapy, only cases for invasive procedures like PTCA or bypass surgery should be considered. It is considered the "gold standard" test and provides the most detailed structural information.

Blood tests can be done to confirm MI

Cardiac enzymes, especially cardiac troponin are useful in distinguishing unstable angina from MI without ST-segment elevation (Antman 2002).

The cardiac enzyme, creatinine kinase, should be tested. The isoenzyme, CK-MB, typically begins to rise within 6 hours of symptom onset, peaks at 18 hours and falls after 24 hours. Serial measurement of total CK and CK-MB should be measured every 6-8 hours for a 24-hour period. Sensitivity is high but specificity is not that good since other causes of myocardial injury will also cause CK-MB elevation.

Cardiac Troponin T and I are located at the contractile apparatus of the myocardium and are highly sensitive to myocardial injury. They provide better sensitivity and specificity for detection of myocardial injury than CK-MB. Troponin T and I are essentially equal in sensitivity and specificities (Olatidoye et al. 1998). They may begin to rise as early as 3 hours but persist for days. On the other hand, the mortality rate was significantly higher in patients with Troponin I > 0.4 mg/ml compared with patients with levels 0.4 mg/ml (Antman et al. 1996). It is usual to check CK-MB and troponin levels simultaneously and serially.

Other differential diagnosis should be investigated accordingly:

- Patients with suspected gastrointestinal pathology such as esophageal reflux can benefit from upper endoscopy, esophageal motility study or 24-hour PH study

- For patients where pulmonary causes are suspected, CXR for patients suspected of pneumothorax. For patients where pulmonary embolism is highly suspected, CXR, ventilation-perfusion scan and/or pulmonary angiography can be considered

- Patients with neuromuscular causes or psychogenic causes do not require further investigation

Pitfalls/Important points to note

The highest priority is generally given to differentiating between chest pain of cardiac and non-cardiac origin. An assessment of the probability of ischaemic heart disease should be made in all patients. Evaluate the cardio-vascular risk factors for all patients who present with chest pain.

Physical examination is usually normal even in serious cardiac cases. No reliable physical signs can be used to determine whether a patient with atypical chest pain has ischaemic heart disease.

For a patient in acute pain with a history highly suggestive of unstable angina, pulmonary embolism or aortic dissection, the decision to immediately hospitalise can be made on the basis of history alone. There is no reason to delay admission.

Description of pain can be greatly influenced by socioeconomic status, education, culture, personality and even gender. Clinical presentation of anginal pain in women especially those aged less than 60 years of age can be very different (Wexler 1999). Chest pain can be absent and the patient may instead present with exertional fatigue, shortness of breath, diaphoresis, arm tingling, jaw discomfort, nausea or indeed abdominal pain—symptoms suggestive of non-anginal pain. This often leads to underdiagnosis or delay in diagnosis of ischaemic heart disease in this particular group of patients.

Diabetes is a major risk factor for early development of ischaemic heart disease. In such patients silent ischaemic changes can occur, i.e. the patient may not suffer from any chest or respiratory symptoms. A normal resting ECG cannot be used as the sole criterion to rule out the presence of ischaemic heart disease. Patients with unstable angina or even an acute myocardial infarct may initially have a normal resting ECG.

Although chest pain may be due to life-threatening ischaemic heart disease, the majority of patients with chest pain have a benign pathology. Family doctors should try to differentiate those with a high probability of ischaemic heart disease whilst we are in the best position to reassure those who have no sinister pathology. It is important not to adopt the practice of defensive medicine as exposure of patients to unnecessary investigations is costly and ethically doubtful.

Management of chest pain

Management of chest pain will depend on subsequent conclusions drawn from history, examination and investigation findings.

Scenario

On further exploration, Mr. Wong did have an episode of similar chest discomfort whilst he was attending his last trail walking training after which he then stopped trail walking, On that occasion, he was walking uphill when he suffered from chest discomfort. He felt that he was dying. His team walkers had to leave him behind. He was alone and felt helpless. He took a rest for around 20 minutes during which time he gradually recovered and decided to walk backward downhill. He was so scared that he did not mention this event even to his wife. Prior to this episode he was in such good health that he seldom went to see a doctor.

Concerning the episodes of chest discomfort associated with lifting heavy objects: The discomfort was mild and without any associated dizziness, sweating or palpitation. No shortness of breath. It was brief and did not occur every time he lifted weights.

Concerning the attack he experienced the night before he attended your surgery: It was after he walked up 5 flights of stairs at home (the lift was out of order). The pain was similar but more severe. It was vaguely defined in location and there was no radiation. However it was associated with shortness of breath and sweating which he thought was normal because of the exercise required to climb the stairs. Once he arrived home, the pain lasted about 5 minutes and subsided with rest. His wife claimed that he looked dreadful and urged him to see a doctor. He thought he was completely well this morning and was reluctant to consult a doctor— he would not have done so if not for his wife.

He claimed that he was a social smoker smoking less than 5 cigarettes per day for the past 20 years. He was not a drinker.

Mr. Wong has 2 elder brothers, 55 years old with hypertension for 5 years and 50 years old in good health. His father died in the war and his mother is 80 years old and bedridden with recurrent stroke.

She has been diagnosed with hypertension and diabetes mellitus since her first stroke at around 70 years old.

Physical examination of Mr. Wong showed his body mass index was 24 (in Asian adults 23–24.9 is considered overweight and at risk), waist circumference 92 cm (in Asian males, normal should be < 90 cm). He claimed that he had gained around 5 kg in recent months with the major decrease in exercise and increased sleep due to tiredness. His blood pressure was 140/95 (rechecked at the end of the consultation it was still 140/95). Heart rate was 72/minute and in sinus rhythm. Other examination was essentially normal. Resting ECG was normal.

His 2 episodes of chest discomfort, the attack associated with trail walking and the one on the day before, were typical of anginal symptoms, whilst the other episodes associated with lifting heavy objects are less conclusive of coronary origin.

With his age > 40 years and typical anginal pain, he has high pre-test probability of IHD. He also has other cardiovascular risk factors: overweight, marginal blood pressure and a smoker.

Initial investigations were done mainly to stratify the cardiovascular risk.

Findings and results

Several blood tests were done:

- Hemoglobin was tested to exclude any underlying anemia, which was normal

- Blood for fasting blood glucose was normal

Lipid profile study showed a total cholesterol (TC) of 5.5 mmol/l and normal triglyceride, HDL and LDL. A "normal" LDL is dependent on whose figures one follows. British Hypertensive Society wants TC < 4 and LDL < 2.

Clinically the diagnosis is stable angina.

Initial management

It might be very difficult for this patient, who has always been healthy, to accept the diagnosis especially when his major expectation of the consultation was to reassure his family that there was nothing wrong. The diagnosis needs to be carefully explained and gently disclosed.

In this case, the explanation would mainly focus on the nature of the diagnosis, the underlying risk factors that increased the cardiovascular risk and also the effect this may have on his daily life, especially with the decrease in exercise tolerance, which limited his trail walking. The family doctor should aim at enhancing a shared understanding with the patient on the nature of the problem. This will greatly assist the formulation of a management plan with the patient and thus improve compliance and control of the symptoms.

As expected, the patient did not react well to the diagnosis. He hoped that further tests could be done to prove that he was not ill. His wife however was very concerned about the diagnosis and hoped he would have early treatment and intervention.

Sublingual glycerol trinitrate (GTN) was prescribed in the first visit whilst awaiting the blood test result. He was advised to take it when required, that is to say whenever he suffered from chest pain or discomfort.

All patients with symptomatic coronary heart disease should be prescribed sublingual GTN and should be educated in its use.

Patients should be advised on how to use this properly and to observe the duration of the pain after taking the sublingual GTN. If pain persists after 3 doses over 15 minutes, patients should promptly refer themselves or be referred to a nearby Accident and Emergency Department.

Patients should also be alerted to the expiry of the drug 8 weeks after opening. Backup supplies should be available when needed (in community pharmacies). Alternatively a GTN sublingual spray could be prescribed as its shelf life can be up to 3 years.

In the subsequent follow-up visit 2 weeks later, the patient had had one mild attack whilst lifting heavy objects during work. He experienced recovery within 3 minutes with the sublingual GTN (in previous episodes he usually needed around 10 minutes rest for complete recovery). He was more convinced of the diagnosis and agreed on collaborative planning to manage his condition.

Further management plan was discussed with him and his wife since it is more effective to encourage the family to modify their lifestyle together and to support him throughout. This has mutual benefit. Not only does it support the patient, but it also reduces the possible risks of cardiovascular disease in the rest of the family.

Further management plans

1. Major objectives of treatment are to prevent death, future cardio-vascular events and to improve symptoms, exercise capacity and quality of life.

2. Management of modifiable risk factors such as weight, smoking habits and increase in total cholesterol.

   - The patient is smoking less than 10 cigarettes a day and nicotine replacement therapy is not needed in principle. He has strong will power and is motivated to quit smoking. He could be referred to smoking cessation class or support group which will enhance the long term success rate of quitting. However with strong support from his family and his non-addictive behaviour, his chances of successfully quitting are high.

   - The patient is overweight. He is encouraged to have regular meals and quantities. He should cut down on simple sugars, food with high fat content and increase fibre intake. Adopting tactics to modify eating behaviour can help, such as drinking a glass of water before each meal, sitting down to eat, taking at least 20 minutes to finish a meal and not skipping meals. Gradual weight loss of 1–2 lb per week is advisable. He should be encouraged to increase aerobic exercise levels within the limits set by his cardiovascular fitness. Diet and exercise together is more effective in preventing weight regain. If necessary, the patient can be referred to a dietitian for advice.

   - The total cholesterol > 5.0 mmol/l. Appropriate dietary measures should be recommended. A limit of total fat intake should be under 30% of calorie intake and preferably rich in monounsaturated fatty acid. Dietary cholesterol should not exceed 300 mg/day. Cholesterol rich foods are restricted. Egg yolk should be limited to no more than 3 per week. The amount of lean meat and fish should be limited to 150–180 g per day. Strict prohibition of seafood is not necessary. Squid and cuttlefish with high cholesterol should be limited and restricted to exchange with egg yolk. Dietary fibre especially soluble fibre should be increased. A dietitian can help to design an individualised diet for the patient. Blood cholesterol should be monitored after 12 weeks of active diet therapy.

3. Blood pressure needs to be monitored on at least one more separate occasion with at least two blood pressure measurements to diagnose hypertension. It was normal (i.e. below 140/85) and it was suggested at our clinic follow up that the patient monitor his blood pressure regularly.

4. Secondary prophylactic treatment should be added. Aspirin 75 mg daily should be used unless contraindicated. Persistent dyspepsia may be treated with antacid, H_2-antagonists or proton pump inhibitor. A history of active peptic ulcer or gastrointestinal bleeding contra-indicates the use of asprin. If helicobactor pyloris is present, eradication therapy should be commenced before starting aspirin. Side-effects should be monitored for in subsequent follow ups.

5. The patient should be monitored for symptoms. Long-term prevention of angina symptoms should be considered. Various researches and random controlled trials (RCT) were done to study the long-term effects of single drug treatment on stable angina. According to the systemic review of Schulpher et al. (1998):

    *   β-blockers: Effective as a single agent in treating angina. RCTs found no significant difference between calcium channel blockers and β-blockers in the frequency of angina attacks, exercise duration, mortality, or non-fatal cardiovascular events at between 6 months and 3 years.
    *   Calcium channel blockers: Effective as a single agent and similar efficacy as β-blockers in RCTs. One RCT found that amlodipine increased exercise duration at 6 months when compared with isosorbide mononitrate. Peripheral oedema is more common as a side-effect of amlodipine.
    *   Nitrates: Effective in treatment of stable angina. One RCT found no significant difference between isosorbide mononitrate and amlodipine in the frequency of angina attacks or in quality of life. The RCT found that headache was more common with isosorbide mononitrate.

- Potassium channel openers: Effective as a single agent.

6. In the local setting, β-blockers are usually the first line of treatment with its lower cost and similar efficacy. Patients who require regular symptomatic treatment should be treated initially with β-blockers (unless contraindicated). Patients should be warned not to stop β-blockers suddenly or allow them to run out. For patients intolerant to β-blockers, alternatives like rate limiting calcium channel blockers, long acting dihydropyridine, nitrate or a potassium channel opening agents can be used. When nitrates are used, sustained release preparation should be used and caution is necessary on allowing a nitrate-free period of 6–8 hours to obviate nitrate tolerance.

7. For patients whose symptoms are not controlled with β-blockers as a single drug, drugs that can be added include isosorbide mononitrate, a long acting dihydropyridine. Caution is needed when diltiazem is used with β-blockers, which needs cardiologist advice. Angio-tensin converting enzyme inhibitiors could be considered in patients with symptoms and signs of heart failure or with chronic left ventricular systolic dysfunction.

8. Referral needs to be considered for:
   - Exercise tolerance test (ETT) for risk stratification
   - Failure to respond to medical treatment (for those who have already had ETT)

   Other indications for referral includes (not in Mr. Wong's case):
   - To confirm or refute the diagnosis when uncertain or with atypical condition
   - Patients who have ejection systolic murmur suggestive of aortic stenosis
   - URGENT referral needed if symptoms are suggestive of unstable angina. For example, anginal pain at rest, pain at minimum exertion like walking 1 flight of stairs at normal pace, pain that is progressing rapidly despite medical treatment (Scottish Intercollegiate Guidelines Network 2006).

9. During follow-up visits in the family medicine clinic, the patient should be monitored for symptom control, compliance to medication and also side-effects of medication. It is equally important to monitor the patient's psychosocial adjustment to the diagnosis of coronary heart disease. This includes effect of the illness on social life and if there is anything to suggest any limitation of exercise tolerance.

Sexual life may be affected by the side-effects of medication as well as by the fear of an attack precipitated by exertion. Depression and panic attacks are not uncommon in patients with ischaemic heart disease. See Chapter 6 for a screening tool for major depression. The family physician, with his continuing relationship with the family, is in a particularly strong position to detect and manage this. Worsening of symptoms can be due to worsening clinical condition or panic attack that can mimic the anginal attack. Emotion is also one known precipitant for triggering an anginal attack.

10. The patient's understanding of the disease, his risk profile and his understanding of how to react when experiencing chest pain or suspected myocardial infarction should be reassessed on subsequent follow ups. Local survey showed that health knowledge of patients with ischaemic heart disease was generally inadequate, especially knowledge of their own risk profile (Leung et al. 2000).

11. When the patient has been stabilised at a specialist clinic, with symptoms under control, and especially for patients with low risk, they should be referred back to the primary care level for further care. A clear management plan should be devised in out patient department to enable family medicine doctors to manage their patients' symptoms and advise on when a patient should be referred back for further management.

12. Screening close relatives of the patient for the possibility of ischaemic heart disease because of the early onset of his coronary heart disease (men under 55 years and women under 65 years)

13. Prognosis: Stable angina is a marker of underlying coronary heart disease.
    - Control of coronary risk factors is important since persistence of these factors exerts a detrimental and additive effect on the prognosis of people with stable angina.
    - People with angina are 2–5 times more likely to develop other manifestations of coronary heart disease than people who do not have angina (Sigurdsson et al. 1995). One population-based study (7,100 men aged 51–59 years at entry) found that people with angina had higher mortality than people with no history of coronary artery disease at baseline (16-year survival rate: 53% with angina vs. 72% without coronary artery disease vs. 34% with a history of myocardial infarction) (Rosengren et al. 1998).

Annual mortality is higher compared with people with no history of coronary artery disease at baseline. Annual mortality is around 1–2% whilst the annual rate of non fatal myocardial infarction is 2–3% (Brunelli et al. 1989; Dargie et al. 1996).

- Poor prognostic factors include more severe symptoms, male sex, abnormal resting ECG, previous myocardial infarction, left ventricular dysfunction, ETT showing widespread and easily provoked ischaemia, significant stenosis of all 3 major coronary arteries or left main coronary artery (Rosengren et al. 1998; Gandhi et al. 1995; Mock et al. 1982).

Summary

The presenting problem of chest pain is common yet very threatening to both patient and doctor because the underlying cause in many instances is potentially lethal especially in the elderly. Therefore it is adamant to treat all sudden onset of chest pain as of cardiac origin until proven otherwise. A careful history is the basis of the diagnosis and patient-centred approach may be the key for some newly diagnosed patients.

References

American College of Emergency Physicians. 1995. "Clinical policy for the initial approach to adults presenting with a chief complaint of chest pain, with no history of trauma". *Annuals of Emergency Medicine*, 25: 274–299.

Antman, E. M. 2002. "Decision making with cardiac troponin tests". *New England Journal of Medicine*, 346 (26): 2002, 2079–2982.

Antman, E. M., Tanasijevic, M. J., Thompson, B., Schactman, M., McCabe, C. H., Cannon, C. P., Fischer, G. A., Fung, A. Y., Thompson, C., Wybenga, D. and Braunwald, E. 1996. "Cardiac-specific Troponin I levels to predict the risk of mortality in patients with acute coronary syndromes". *New England Journal of Medicine*, 335: 1342–1349.

Brunelli, C., Cristofani, R. and L'Abbate, A. 1989. "Long-term survival in medically treated patients with ischaemic heart disease and prognostic importance of clinical and echocardiographic data". *European Heart Journal*, 10: 292–303.

Dargie, H. J., Ford, I. and Fox, K. M. 1996. "Total Ischaemic Burden European

Trial (TIBET). Effects of ischaemia and treatment with atenolol, nifedipine SR and their combination on outcome in patients with chronic stable angina". *European Heart Journal*, 17: 104–112.

Diamond, G. A. and Forrester, J. S. 1979. "Analysis of probability as an aid in the clinical diagnosis of coronary-artery disease". *New England Journal of Medicine*, 300: 1350.

Ebell, M. H. 2001. *Evidence-based Diagnosis: A Handbook of Clinical Prediction Rules*. New York: Springer-Verlag.

Fesmire, F. M., Percy, R. F., Bardoner, J. B.,Wharton, D. R. and Calhoun, F. B. 1998. "Usefulness of automated serial 12 lead ECG monitoring during the initial emergency department evaluation of patients with chest pain". *Annals of Emergency Medicine*, 31 (1): 3–11.

Gandhi, M. M., Lampe, F. C. and Wood, D. A. 1995. "Incidence, clinical characteristics and short-term prognosis of angina pectoris". *British Heart Journal*, 73: 193–198.

Garber, A. M. and Solomon, N. A. 1999. "Cost effectiveness of alternative test strategies for the diagnosis of coronary artery disease". *Annals of Internal Medicine*, 130: 719.

Kuntz, K. M., Fleischmann, K. E., Hunink, M. G. M. and Douglas, P. S. 1999. "Cost effectiveness of diagnostic strategies for patients with chest pain". *Annuals of Internal Medicine*, 130: 709.

Leung, K. F., Chan, W. K., Law, K. F. and Yue, C. S. 2000. "Health knowledge of patients with ischaemic heart disease: How much do they know? How do they react to chest pain and suspected myocardial infarction?" *Hong Kong Practitioner*, 22: 219–225.

Mock, M. B., Ringqvist, I., Fisher, L. D., Davis, K. B., Chaitman, B. R., Kouchoukos, N. T., Kaiser, G. C., Alderman, E., Ryan, T. J., Russell, R. O., Mullin, S., Fray, D. and Killip, T. 1982. "Survival of medically treated patients in the Coronary Artery Surgery Study (CASS) registry". *Circulation*, 66: 562–568.

Morrow, D. A., Antman, E. M., Charlesworth, A., Cairus, R., Murphy, S. A., de Lemos, J. A., Giugliano, R. P., McCabe, C. H. and Braunwald, E. 2000. "TIMI risk score for ST elevation myocardial infarction: A convenient bedside, clinical score for risk assessment at presentation: An intravenous nPA for treatment of infarcting myocardium early II trial substudy". *Circulation*, 102 (17): 2031–2037.

Olatidoye, A. G., Wu, A. H., Feng, Y. J. and Waters, D. 1998. "Prognostic role of Troponin T versus Troponin I in unstable angina pectoris for cardiac events with meta-angina pectoris for cardiac events with meta-analysis comparing published studies". *American Journal of Cardiology*, 81: 1405–1410.

Rosengren, A., Wilhelmsen, L., Hagman, M. and Wedel, H. 1998. "Natural history of myocardial infarction and angina pectoris in a general population sample of middle aged men: A 16-year follow-up of the Primary Prevention Study, Goteborg, Sweden". *Journal of Internal Medicine*, 244: 495–505.

Sabatine, M. S., McCabe, C. H., Morrow, D. A., Giugliano, R. P., de Lemos, J. A., Cohen, M., Antman, E. M. and Braunwald, E. 2002. "Identification of patients at high risk for death and cardiac ischemic events after hospital discharge". *American Heart Journal*, 143 (6): 966–970.

Schulpher, M., Petticrew, M., Kelland, J. L., Elliott, R. A., Holdrights, D. R. and Buxton, M. J. 1998. "Resource allocation in chronic stable angina: A systematic review of the effectiveness, costs and cost-effectiveness of alternative interventions". *Health Technology Assess*, 2 (10): i–iv, 1–176.

Scottish Intercollegiate Guidelines Network (SIGN). "Guideline on management of stable angina". Retrieved 23 January, 2006, from http://www.sign.ac.uk/guidelines/published/index.html.

Sigurdsson, E., Sigfusson, N., Agnarsson, U., Sigvaldason, H. and Thorgeirsson, G. 1995. "Long-term prognosis of different forms of coronary heart disease: The Reykjavik Study". *International Journal of Epidemiology*, 24: 58–68.

Wexler, L. 1999. "Studies of acute coronary syndromes in women—lessons for everyone". *New England Journal of Medicine*, 341: 275.

Chapter 13

Abdominal Symptoms: Dyspepsia or Indigestion

◆ Samuel Y. S. WONG ◆

Scenario

A 50-year-old executive comes to the family medicine clinic with complaints of discomfort in the stomach for several weeks. On questioning, you understand that his discomfort originates from the epigastric region with occasional nausea, excessive belching and feeling of slow digestion. He smokes a pack of cigarettes a day and drinks wine a few times with dinner per week. The discomfort usually bothers him in the morning but has never awakened him at night.

What are the likely diagnoses and how do you proceed to make a final diagnosis?

Symptoms related to the dysfunction of the upper gastrointestinal (GI) tract—such as upper abdominal pain or discomfort may also include symptoms of fullness, bloating, distension, heartburn, waterbrash, nausea and vomiting. An organic cause can be found in 40% of patients with dyspeptic symptoms.

The most likely causes

- Gastro-duodenal ulcer
- Gastro-oesophageal reflux disease

    In up to 60% of cases, no cause can be identified and is considered to be idiopathic (functional, e.g. irritable bowel syndrome or non-ulcer dyspepsia).

The important possibility that (may) need to be excluded

• Gastric cancer

Irritable bowel syndrome

In 1991 an international panel of clinical investigators developed a classification of functional gastrointestinal disorders (Talley et al. 1991), including dyspepsia, which was recently updated at the Rome II Consensus Conference (Talley et al. 1999). The following definition for functional dyspepsia was recommended: "Twelve weeks or more (within the last 12 months) of persistent or recurrent dyspepsia and evidence that organic disease likely to explain the symptoms is absent (including at upper endoscopy)."

Non-ulcer (functional) dyspepsia can be subcategorised into:

1. Ulcer-like: characterised by upper abdominal pain

2. Reflux-like: characterised by heartburn, regurgitation or both

3. Dysmotility-like: characterised by symptoms of nausea, vomiting, early satiety, and abdominal bloating or distention

However the usefulness of this subclassification based on symptoms is questionable as cases tend to overlap among the subtypes. Thus the subcategorisation has poor predictive value when the same patient undergoes endoscopy.

Pre-investigation diagnosis

According to the Canadian Medical Association guideline for "an evidence-based approach to the management of un-investigated dyspepsia in the era of Helicobacter pylori (H. pylori)" (*Canadian Medical Association Journal* 2000), there are 5 key decision points in the clinical management.

1. *Identification of patients with other possible causes of dyspeptic symptoms*

Careful history taking and physical examination should identify patients for whom it is necessary to exclude cardiac (associated with exercise, duration of symptoms, shortness of breath, palpitations, diaphoresis, cardiac risk factors, etc.), hepatobiliary (location of pain, quality of pain, radiation, nausea or vomiting) and other non-gastrointestinal origins of the presenting dyspeptic symptoms (medication history: use of new medication, e.g. antidepressants, etc.; lifestyle history: smoking, alcohol use). However for dyspepsia, the positive predictive value of symptoms for ulcer or cancer remains disappointing. The role of the physical examination, in terms of adding to diagnostic precision, is also limited (Fisher et al. 1998) although patients may feel the physician's physical examination is important.

2. *Older patients and patients with alarming features*

Older patients and patients with alarming features have a higher risk for organic causes of dyspepsia including cancer (< 2%) and ulcer. Retrospective studies showed that most young patients with gastric or oesophageal cancer presented with at least one alarming feature (see below). In large epidemiological studies in the West it was shown that gastric and oesophageal cancers were rarely a cause of dyspeptic symptoms in younger patients. In these studies, no cases of either cancer were reported in any patient younger than 45 years of age (Williams et al. 1988; Hallissey et al. 1990). Indeed, the age threshold for a recommendation for prompt endoscopy should be driven by the prevalence of gastric and oesophageal cancer in the population in which one practises, and this may vary from country to country (age 45 for Americans, 50 for Canadians). Some evidence in Hong Kong suggests that the threshold may need to be lowered.

In a large local study in patients with dyspepsia with and without alarming features, 17.4% of patients in the low-risk group (those 45 years of age or younger without alarming features) were found to have cancer whereas in Western studies almost none of the patients in this group had cancer (Sung et al. 2001).

Alarming features and their applications (VBAD):

- Age > 45
- Vomiting (V)
- Bleeding/Anaemia (B)
- Abdominal mass/Unexplained weight loss (A)
- Dysphagia (D)

3. *Patients who use non-steroidal anti-inflammatory drugs (NSAIDs)*

Chronic users of NSAIDs including aspirin are associated with increased risk of gastric and duodenal ulcers. The prevalence of peptic ulcers in people who use NSAIDs regularly is between 10% and 30% (relative risk of 3 times that of non-users). NSAIDs are responsible for most non-H. pylori negative ulcers.

4. *Identification of patients with dominant symptoms of heartburn or acid regurgitation or both*

Studies showed that when heartburn ("a burning feeling arising from the stomach or lower chest toward the neck") or acid regurgitation are the dominant symptoms, they will have a high specificity (89% and 95% respectively) for gastro-oesophageal reflux disease (GORD). One important point to note is that most patients with GORD do not have macroscopic oesophagitis and therefore have endoscopy-negative reflux disease.

5. *Helicobacter pylori "test-and-treat" strategy for patients with uninvestigated dyspepsia without alarming features*

A test-and-treat strategy is recommended for uninvestigated dyspepsia in younger patients in Western countries (aged 45 years or less) who have no alarming features. The main options include the following:

- A trial of empiric (antisecretory or prokinetic) therapy, with investigation reserved for symptomatic failures

- Diagnostic evaluation for all (preferably endoscopy), with treatment based on the findings

- Non-invasive testing for H. pylori followed by eradication therapy for patients with positive results ("test-and-treat")

- Non-invasive testing for H. pylori followed by endoscopy for patients with positive results

 There is accumulating evidence that the test-and-treat approach is both safe and cost-effective, especially where the prevalence of peptic ulcer disease and H. pylori infection are high. Although a "test-and-treat" strategy for H. pylori infection has been recommended in Europe and North America as safe and cost-effective for management of patients with dyspepsia, the applicability of such a strategy in Hong Kong awaits further studies.

H. pylori is associated with peptic ulcer disease, gastric cancer, non-ulcer dyspepsia, oesophagitis and other conditions ranging from cardiovascular disease to haematological malignancy. Tests for H. pylori include serology, urea breath test, Clo-test and faecal antigen test.

Suggested investigations

Anyone with "red flag" features should be referred for urgent endoscopy. For those who do not have any alarming features but are taking NSAIDs, the NSAIDs should be stopped and symptoms be monitored closely. Those who are taking NSAIDs and are aged under 45 should be tested for H. pylori with eradication therapy if results are positive. Those who are older than 45 without past history of gastric ulcer or duodenal ulcer disease should have endoscopy.

Those with history of duodenal ulcer and symptomatic or requiring long-term acid suppressive therapy should be treated without testing.

Red flag features (Talley and Vakil 2005):

1. Age of onset cut-off
    a. Current age cut-off: age over 45–56 years
    b. Recent literature suggests adjusting based on gender
        i. Age over 35 years in men
        ii. Age over 56 years in women

2. Dysphagia

3. Anorexia or early satiety

4. Persistent vomiting

5. Jaundice

6. Abnormality in physical examination findings

7. Family history of gastric cancer
    a. More common in non-Caucasian

8. Prior peptic ulcer disease history

9. Unexplained weight loss
    a. Weight loss > 3 kg or 6.5 pounds
    b. Weight loss > 10% of body weight

10. Signs of significant gastrointestinal bleeding
    a. Anaemia
    b. Rectal bleeding or melena

Findings and results

The man was referred to have an endoscopy after he had consulted a gastroenterologist. His biopsy result showed positive H. pylori with gastritis. You then decided to treat him.

Management of abdominal symptoms

Eradication therapy

- Combinations of proton pump inhibitor (PPI), bismuth, ranitidine, and one or more antibiotics are used. All have 10–20% failure rate
- PPI + clarithromycin + either amoxicillin or metronidazole—1 week (90–95% success)
- PPI + amoxicillin + metronidazole—2 weeks (80–85%)
- Bismuth + metronidaxole + tetracycline—2 weeks
- Other combinations
- Check eradication post-treatment by urea breath test or faecal antigen test
- Compliance is an important predictor of success

Long-term care

Long-term care in dyspepsia relates to the long-term management of GORD. Family doctors need to be aware that GORD can lead to major complications and acid reflux is a risk factor for the development of adenocarcinoma of the oesophagus. Effective acid suppression in reflux disease is important, and a step down approach (beginning with maximum therapy and reducing dosage to a level at which symptoms are controlled) is most appropriate. Lifestyle modification in patients to reduce risk, i.e. smoking and alcohol drinking habits, and weight reduction is also important.

Summary

• Taking relevant gastrointestinal history and especially knowing the alarming features and their use in local population

• Importance of treating H. pylori and the recommended approach for test-and-treat strategies

References

Fisher, R. S. and Parkman, H. P. 1998. "Current concepts: Management of nonulcer dyspepsia". *New England Journal of Medicine*, 339 (19): 1376–1381.

Hallissey, M. T., Allum, W. H., Jewkes, A. G., Ellis, D. J. and Fielding, J. W. L. 1990. "Early detection of gastric cancer". *British Medical Journal*, 301: 513–515.

Hu, W. H. C., Wong, W. M., Lam, C. L. K., Lam, K. F., Hui, W. M., Lai, K. C., Xia, H. X. H., Lam, S. K. and Wong, B. C. Y. 2002. "Anxiety but not depression determines health care-seeking behavior in Chinese patients with dyspepsia and irritable bowel syndrome: A population based study". *Alimentary Pharmacology and Therapeutics*, 16: 2081–2088.

Lu, C. L., Lang, H. C., Chang, F. Y., Chen, C. Y., Luo, J. C., Wang, S. S. and Lee, S. D. 2005. "Prevalence and health/social impacts of functional dyspepsia in Taiwan: A study based on Rome criteria questionnaire survey assisted by endoscopic exclusion among a physical check-up population". *Scandinavian Journal of Gastroenterology*, 40 (4): 402–411.

Sung, J. J., Lao, W. C., Lai, M. S., Li, T. H., Chan, F. K., Wu, J. C., Leung, V. K., Luk, Y. W., Kung, N. N., Ching, J. Y., Leung, W. K., Lau, J. and Chung, S. J. 2001. "Incidence of gastroesophageal malignancy in patients with dyspepsia in Hong Kong: Implications for screening strategies". *Gastrointestinal Endoscopy*, 54: 454–458.

Talley, N. J., Colin-Jones, D., Koch, K. L., Koch, M., Nyren, O. and Stanghellini, V. 1991. "Functional dyspepsia: A classification with guidelines for diagnosis and management". *Gastroenterology International*, (4): 145–160.

Talley, N. J., Stanghellini, V., Heading, R., Koch, K. L., Malagelada, J. R. and Tytgat, G. N. J. 1999. "Functional gastroduodenal disorders". *Gut*, 45(12) (Supp. 12): 137–142.

Talley, N. J. and Vakil, N. 2005. "Guidelines for the management of dyspepsia". *American Journal of Gastroenterology*, 100: 2324–2337.

Van Zanten, S. J. O., Flook, N., Chiba, N., Armstrong, D., Barkun, A., Bradette, M., Thomson, A., Bursey, F., Blackshaw, P., Frai, D., Sinclair, P. and the Canadian Dyspepsia Working Group. 2000. "An evidence-based approach to the management of uninvestigated dyspepsia in the era of Helicobacter pylori". *Canadian Medical Association Journal*, 162 (12) (Supp.): 3–23.

Williams, B., Luckas, M., Ellingham, J. H. M., Dain, A. and Wicks, A. C. B. 1988. "Do young patients with dyspepsia need investigation?" *Lancet*, 2: 1349–1351.

Chapter 14

Dizziness

◆ Martin LINDSAY ◆

Scenario

A 77-year-old lady comes to see you with a 4-week history of giddiness.

What are the likely diagnoses and how do you proceed to make a final diagnosis?

Why does dizziness cause all family doctors' hearts to sink? The initial dilemma is "What does the patient mean by dizziness?" It is a totally non-specific term. It could be interpreted as anything from syncope to drowsiness to vertigo to giddiness (and a variety of other terms too). The next quandary lies in the fact that it is an all too common presentation with numerous possible causes (many of a serious nature). Consequently, the doctors are concerned that they do not miss one of those life-threatening diagnoses from one of those long lists of possibilities. The final catch is that despite the doctors knowing that nothing will be found seriously wrong in the vast majority of patients, many questions still have to be asked and a full examination has to be made.

Classifying by systems

The first way is by subdividing into systemic categories such as:

1. Ear (inner and middle)
2. Cardiovascular

3. Cervical spine
4. Brain
5. Anxiety-hyperventilation
6. Vaso-vagal
7. Drug
8. Others

   Then take the possible diagnoses in each system.

Inner ear

- Acoustic neuroma

Middle ear

- Otitis media/externa including Ramsay-Hunt Syndrome
- Wax
- Auditory tube dysfunction

Cardiovascular

- Anaemia
- Arrhythmias
- Aortic stenosis
- Hypertension or hypotension

Cervical spine

- Cervical spondylosis causing vertebro-basilar insufficiency (VBI)

Brain

- Transient ischaemic attack (TIA)/Cerebro-vascular accident (CVA)
- Any space-occupying lesion, e.g. tumours, abscesses
- Multiple sclerosis

Drug

- Alcohol
- Ototoxic drugs, e.g. aspirin/NSAIDs, gentamycin, antidepressants, antihypertensives, antipsychotics and antiepiletics

Others

- Hypoglycaemia
- Psychogenic

Classifying by symptoms

Vertigo

This is the sensation that oneself or one's surroundings are rotating/ spinning even though the person concerned is stationary.

Vertigo is subdivided into central and peripheral causes. The central causes of vertigo include:

- Brainstem, i.e. VBI or TIA/CVA
- Cerebro-pontine angle tumours
- Migraine
- Multiple sclerosis
- Epilepsy
- Cerebellar degeneration

The peripheral causes of vertigo include:

Labyrinthine involvement

- Meniere's disease (paroxysmal attacks of vertigo plus progressive deafness and tinnitus)
- Viral labyrinthitis (acute vertigo plus deafness and tinnitus)
- Benign positional vertigo
- Drugs
- Trauma
- Otitis media

Eighth nerve involvement

- Acoustic neuroma
- Drugs
- Vestibular neuronitis (acute vertigo only)
- Perilymph fistula
- Glomus tumour
- Peripheral vestibular dysfunction

Syncope

This is a loss of consciousness.

Cardiovascular causes

*   Anaemia
*   Hypertension
*   Postural hypotension
*   Vaso-vagal
*   TIA/CVA
*   Arrhythmia
*   Aortic stenosis

Others

*   Anxiety-hyperventilation
*   Head injury
*   Drugs

Giddiness

A non-specific term. Sensation of ill-defined light-headedness. Symptoms are as for syncope, plus:

*   Wax
*   Cervical spondylosis
*   Auditory tube dysfunction

Note these lists are not exhaustive.

You can now begin to appreciate the family doctors' predicament. Both ways of categorising the problems are useful, but they are cumbersome.

Classifying by a combination of likelihood and system involved

To a degree this is age-related. For example, the elderly are more likely to have wax in their ears causing dizziness, whilst young women who skip breakfast can become hypoglycaemic around mid-morning or have a vaso-vagal attack in hot, stuffy places.

The most likely causes (subdivided into age-related risks)

Ear

- Otitis media/externa including Ramsay-Hunt Syndrome
- Auditory tube dysfunction
- Viral labyrinthitis or neuronitis
- Benign paroxysmal positional vertigo
- Wax*
- Meniere's disease*

Cardiovascular

- Anaemia
- Arrhythmias*
- Postural hypotension*
- Hypertension

Neck

- Cervical spondylosis*/VBI*

Others

- Drugs including alcohol
- Anxiety-hyperventilation

Especially the young (usually women)

- Vaso-vagal
- Hypoglycaemia

* Especially among the elderly

The important possibilities that (may) need to be excluded

- Space-occupying lesions including acoustic neuroma and other cancers, abscesses
- Aortic stenosis
- Myocardial infarction
- CVA/TIA

The rare or unusual possibilities

- Head injuries (unless previously known)
- Cerebellar degeneration

- Epilepsy
- Multiple sclerosis
- Migraine
- Perilymph fistula

Symptoms pattern

Whatever the cause of the dizziness, the following questions are always important to elucidate the cause.

- Timing: frequency; onset, duration; time of day
- What is the person doing at time of onset?
- Any associated symptoms?

Specific questions to ask that may help

- *Is this vertigo and if so how long does it last?*
  This is the first question. If there is vertigo, then the majority of the potential causes are removed. So ask if the patient has a sensation of movement with one of those episodes.

  Then you can ask the subsequent questions about any associated features, what the person is doing at the time of onset, and the timing.

- *Any history of an upper respiratory tract infection?*
  If yes the possibilities include viral neuronitis, viral labyrinthitis or auditory tube dysfunction. (The usual history is for the vertigo to be present for several days and then begin to improve followed by full recovery over the subsequent few weeks. However in primary care, patients invariable present within 48 hours of the onset of vertigo. Thus it is not always possible to be 100% sure of the final diagnosis but this may make it more likely.)

- *How severe is the vertigo?*
  Very severe = viral neuronitis or viral labyrinthitis
  (If the vertigo is associated with tinnitus and deafness it is more likely to be viral labyrinthitis.)
  Mild = auditory tube dysfunction

- *Any headaches?*
  Migraine (especially if there is a past or family history)
- *Is it associated with head movements?*
  Paroxysmal benign positional vertigo/VBI
- *Has the vertigo been present for several weeks and is not improving?*
  Meniere's disease, drug-induced, brain tumours (uncommon)

If there is no vertigo

Again, the same questions need to be asked:

- Timing: frequency; onset and duration; time of day
- What is the person doing at time of onset?
- Any associated symptoms?

At this point it might be easier to consider the age/probability/system list to help recall the possibilities so that it is a bit easier not to forget the potential causes.

Table 14.1 Taking the questions system by system

Symptoms	Cause(s)
ENT	
Deafness	Wax, otitis media/externa including Ramsay-Hunt Syndrome, auditory tube dysfunction or perilymph fistula
Tinnitus	Meniere's disease, auditory tube dysfunction, CPA tumour (see below)
Otalgia or a feeling of fullness in the ear	Wax, otitis media/externa including Ramsay-Hunt Syndrome or auditory tube dysfunction
Discharge from the ear	Otitis externa
Cardiovascular	
Symptoms on standing up	Postural hypotension

Symptoms	Cause(s)
Palpitations	Arrhythmia
History of cardiovascular disease	Hypertension, ischaemic heart or vascular disease
Irregular pulse	Arrhythmia
Exertional chest pains	Aortic stenosis, ischaemic heart disease including myocardial infarction
Short of breath, fatigue	Anaemia, anxiety-hyperventilation, aortic stenosis
Feeling flushed in face, vision going black from periphery inwards, etc.	Vaso-vagal

Neck

Neck problems	Cervical spondylosis/VBI

Neurological

Anything to suggest a fit	Epilepsy
Throbbing headaches	Migraine
Neurological symptoms e.g. cranial nerve palsies, hemiparesis, hemisensory loss or impaired consciousness	Space-occupying lesions incl. acoustic neuroma & other cancers, abscesses, CVA/TIA or multiple sclerosis
Incoordination or dysarthria	Cerebellar degeneration or lesion
Head injuries	Brain damage
Cerebellopontine angle tumour	Facial numbness, cerebellar incoordination, tinnitus, dysarthria
Eighth cranial nerve palsy	Associated facial weakness
Anxiety/Depression	Hyperventilation and frontal lobe tumours

Others

Missed breakfast	Hypoglycaemia
Psychogenic	Anxiety/Depression

Drug history

Especially ototoxic drugs including:

Alcohol	Gentamycin	Antihypertensives	Antiepiletics
Aspirin/NSAI	Antidepressants	Antipsychotics	

Scenario

A 77-year-old lady comes to see you with a 4-week history of giddiness. She says that she comes over feeling dizzy at no particular time of day. She is slightly deaf but has been so for some time. There has been no recent change to her deafness. No other ENT symptoms. The episodes last up to 10 minutes but are not associated with loss of consciousness, headache, head movements, standing or other neurological symptoms. Psychiatric assessment failed to show evidence of dementia or anxiety-depression. She has a history of folate deficient anaemia due to poor diet but has been taking her folic acid for some time but no other medication. No other past history of note. She lives alone in a warden-controlled flat (i.e. her flat is one of several in a block of flats. A warden is in attendance who could visit in an emergency. However they could not supervise a patient 24 hours a day).

A working diagnosis

Based on the history alone, the most likely causes are as follows:

- Wax
- Anaemia
- Arrhythmia
- Hypertension
- Aortic stenosis
- Vaso-vagal
- Cervical spondylosis/VBI
- TIA

Examination

This is very much governed by the history. The following systems should be examined: ear, nose and throat, cardiovascular, cranial nerves, neurological and the neck.

More specifically always consider performing the following:

- ENT: Otoscopy; tuning fork tests; Hallpike's manoeuvre
- Cranial nerves: Especially nerves 5 to 7 as they pass through the cerebro-pontine angle; eye movements looking for

- Neurology: nystagmus or patient complaining of diplopia; fundoscopy

- Neurology: Especially cereballar functions such as finger-nose test; heel-shin test; Romberg's test

- Cardiovascular: Blood pressure both sitting and standing; heart sounds; carotid bruits; pulse rhythm and rate

- Neck: Check not only for full movement but also if any particular movement creates the symptoms the patient is complaining of

Scenario

On examination the following were the findings:

- ENT: Nil abnormal found. In particular there was no wax

- Cranial nerves: Nil abnormal

- Neurology: Nil abnormal

- Cardiovascular: BP sitting and standing was normal. Heart sounds were also normal. No carotid bruits

- Neck: Some limited range of movement in all directions but none of the movements created any dizziness symptoms

Investigations

Just like the examination, this is very much dependent on the history and the clinical findings. The following are all possibilities:

Investigation	Reason
FBC	Anaemia
ESR	Non specific screen
Random glucose	Hypoglycaemia/Diabetes mellitus
Resting ECG	Arrhythmias
Cervical spine X-ray	Cervical spondylosis—however most elderly patients have X-ray changes compatible with this. Without symptoms provoked by movement it is unlikely to be helpful

Second line investigation	Reason
24-hour ECG (2nd line—if continue to be dizzy and no other pathology found)	Arrhythmias
Echocardiogram (ditto)	Valvular disease including aetiology of TIAs
Exercise ECG (ditto)	Ischaemic heart disease
Carotid doppler	Carotid artery stenosis
Tilt-table test	Autonomic neuropathy
CT scan	Suspected brain lesions
MRI	Suspected brain lesions
EEG	Epilepsy
Audiology	To determine if conductive or sensori-neural deafness
Chest X-ray	Only if considering that a tumour is likely cause

Specific to this scenario

Investigation	Reason
FBC	History of anaemia
RBC folate	History of folate deficiency anaemia (RBC folate is far more accurate than serum folate to establish if there is folate deficiency)
ESR	Non specific screen
Glucose	Screen for hypoglycaemia and diabetes
Resting ECG	Even though nil abnormal on examination. It is an easy non invasive investigation

Findings and results

All the results came back as normal. Thus the post-investigatory differential diagnoses list is now:

- Arrhythmia
- Anxiety-hyperventilation
- Vaso-vagal attack
- TIA

Management of dizziness

Initial management

With an unclear diagnosis and two of the possibilities being of a serious nature, the family doctor has only one option, that is, to refer the patient to the appropriate specialist. In this case, doctors for the elderly (geriatricians). She was also prescribed a low dose aspirin (in case of TIA) and for symptomatic relief, an anti-emetic used to treat vertigo (e.g. prochlorperazine).

The hospital specialist arranged for 24-hour ECG (results: normal), CT scan (normal), tilt-table test (normal), audiological assessment by a different specialist (normal), echocardiogram (normal), a neurological opinion (including EEG—normal). Thus the diagnosis was never established. She continued on symptomatic treatment.

Follow-up management

However over a period of several months, the cause became obvious. She started to telephone in the middle of the night asking for an emergency visit. The doctors called—nothing wrong could be found. Then during the day, she started doing the same. Instead of visiting, the doctors then started to telephone her back. After a very brief conversation she felt much better.

The diagnosis was one of loneliness. Unfortunately she still refused to move to an old age home where she could meet more people and have greater support. She continues to telephone whenever she is lonely despite the given suggestions.

Summary

You have now spent some considerable time reading all these pages on dizziness, trying to work out (we hope) the cause of this patient's symptoms. Having considered all those serious causes (and less serious causes too), you (just like family doctors) find that despite all your good intentions and hard work there is no physical cause after all. Frustrating, isn't it? But at least you will not be troubled by this patient in the middle of the night any more!

Chapter 15

Headaches

◆ Martin LINDSAY ◆

Scenario

Ms. A is a 28-year-old single parent with two children aged 2 and 6. She comes to see you complaining of headaches for the last 6 months.

What are the likely diagnoses and how do you proceed to make a final diagnosis?

The most likely causes

- Tension headaches
- Migraines
- Anxiety/Depression, i.e. presenting with a headache
- Infections, e.g. influenza/upper respiratory tract infection
- Referred from neck
  - ❖ Levator scapulae syndrome as part of a stress disorder and therefore distinct from depression, or
  - ❖ Cervical spondylosis—not likely in this age group but would be if much older or possibly if she had sustained a serious whiplash injury in the past

The important possibilities that (may) need to be excluded

- Tumours (including brain tumours)

- Sub-arachnoid haemorrhage (SAH)
- Severe or malignant hypertension
- Benign-intercranial hypertension
- Meningitis
- Temporal arteritis

The rare or unusual possibilities

- Cluster headache
- Post-coital headaches
- ENT aetiology, e.g. sinusitis, otitis media
- Ophthalmic, e.g. glaucoma
- Dental
- Analgesia-induced headache
- Other drugs causing headaches, e.g. anti hypertensives, hormonal contraceptives, etc.
- Excessive caffeine, e.g. coffee, tea, cola drinks
- Ice-cream headache

What questions do you ask?

Remember your "Most Likely and Important Lists". It is *essential* to get a complete and accurate history as in the vast majority of patients with headaches, the diagnosis is made solely from the history. Examination is invariably normal in headache patients.

The questions

- Site of headache
- Duration
- Frequency
- Radiation
- Type of pain, e.g. throbbing, aching, pounding, stabbing, pressure, etc.
- Associated features, e.g. photophobia
- Precipitating features
- Relieving features
- Family history of headaches
- Past history of headaches

The sinister questions

- No previous history of headaches
- Systemic illness including pyrexia
- Weight loss
- Severe and acute onset
- Personality change, e.g. depression, forgetful, aggression, etc.
- Other neurological symptoms such as long-tract or focal symptoms
- Visual symptoms
- Loss of consciousness or fits
- Repeated vomiting

Symptoms pattern

As already mentioned, the answer to some of these questions can give a very clear lead as to the cause of the headache.

For example, the type of pain: Throbbing headaches imply migraine. Pressure or weight on top of the head or vice-like implies tension headaches. Pain radiating up the back of the neck to the vault from the shoulders implies levator scapulae syndrome causing a tension type headache (usually stress-related).

Other answers may not give a clear lead. For example, duration: A headache lasting 4 hours may be either migraine or a tension headache. Without further information it would be impossible to know. On the other hand, a headache persisting for more than 24 hours excludes a tension headache and many of the rare or unusual causes.

Relieving features—headache improves while lying down in a quiet dark room is classical of a migraine but could also be effective for someone with a severe tension headache.

Again this emphasises the necessity for a complete and accurate history.

Specific questions to ask that may help

Obviously, at some point in the consultation it may well be worthwhile asking the sinister questions. However do realise that the important causes of headaches are not at all common. For example, in 17 years of practice and a list size of some 12,000 patients, I have only seen 2 cases of sub-arachnoid haemorrhage as a cause of headache. I have never seen tumours or meningitis solely presenting as a headache, and never seen severe or malignant hypertension or benign-intercranial hypertension at all. (The incidence of SAH, for example, is 6 per 100,000 patients years [van Gijn and Rinkel 2001]. In terms of an average family practice of 2,400 people [1,000 patients between 45 and 84 years of age], 4 patients will have a stroke per annum whilst one will have a TIA. Intracerebral haemorrhage will occur about twice every 3 years, and sub-arachnoid haemorrhage once every 8 years.)

Precipitating features may also be helpful in not only delineating the type of headache but also its remedy. For example, certain foods may cause migraine. The classic examples are cheese, red wine and chocolate. On the other hand, ice cream (or indeed any ice-cold food or drink) might conceivably cause an "ice-cream headache"—these are typically an intense stabbing pain in the head that lasts 30–60 seconds. Either way, by not taking these substances the patient will not get any headaches.

Do check to see if there is anything to suggest a mental health problem such as stress, anxiety or depression. If in doubt it is pretty reasonable to use the "Screening Tool for Major Depression", i.e.

During the past month have you often been bothered by:

* Feeling down, depressed or hopeless?
* Little interest or pleasure in doing things?

Followed by "Is this something with which you would like help?"

A family history of migraine is a helpful pointer. Do not forget about abdominal migraine either. Do ask about recurrent abdominal pain in childhood, as the adult may not have been told about the cause of this as a child.

The periodicity can also give helpful clues:

- Periodic: migraine, tension headaches, cervical spondylosis and depression
- Persistent   tension headaches, infections (e.g. viral illness, meningitis), tumours, depression, temporal arteritis, raised intra-cranial pressure

The speed of onset provides yet other clues:

- Acute (immediate) onset:
  Sub-arachnoid haemorrhage, coitus headaches, ice-cream headaches, cluster headaches
- Sub-acute onset, i.e. starts over a period of minutes:
  Migraine (as usually have prodromal symptoms and possibly aura), infections (e.g. viral illness, meningitis) as again associated with other symptoms initially, tension headaches, cervical spondylosis
- Chronic onset, i.e. very slow build up over a period of hours:
  Migraine (as usually have prodromal symptoms and possibly aura)

Site of the headache:

- Occipital:
  Hypertension, from neck (levator scapulae syndrome or cervical spondylosis), raised intra-cranial pressure, sub-arachnoid haemorrhage
- From neck, over vault to front:
  Levator scapulae syndrome or cervical spondylosis
- Unilateral:
  Migraine (though may become bilateral)
- Bilateral:
  Tension headaches, analgesic headaches
- Vault-/Band-like:
  Tension headache (the distribution is due to tension of the muscles inserting into the cranium—this pulls on the peri-osteum, thus creating pain, and thus the distribution is along the lines of muscle insertion)
- Frontal:
  Sinusitis or cluster headaches
- Forehead/Temples:
  Temporal arteritis, migraine

By far the two commonest types of headaches encountered in family medicine are tension headache and migraine. A synopsis of both follows.

Tension headaches

Features:

- Mild to moderate in severity
- Symptoms typically get worse during the day
- Photophobia, phonophobia and nausea may occur
- Bilateral in 90%
- Often felt as a pressure or constriction or band-like
- There is no aura
- Not accompanied by significant systemic upset or neurological deficits

Tension-type headaches

- Episodic tension-type headache
- Chronic tension-type headache
  - ❖ Pain for more than 15 days in the month
  - ❖ May have chronic daily headaches
  - ❖ Precipitated by stress, work, menstruation, etc.
  - ❖ Recognised as a "normal headache"

Migraines

Features:
- Lasting 4–72 hours

According to the Migraine Action Association UK and the "Simplified diagnostic criteria for migraine" (after Goadsby and Olesen [1996] and adapted from the International Headache Society), two of the following are also features of migraines:

- Unilateral pain
- Throbbing quality
- Aggravated by movement
- Moderate/Severe pain

  And one of the following:

- Nausea/Vomiting
- Photo- or phono-phobia

Migraine phases

There are four phases:

1. Prodromal
2. Aura
3. Headache
4. Resolution

1. Prodromal

These are the commonest feelings but the list is not exhaustive:

- Mood changes
- Coldness or warmth
- Anorexia or increased appetite
- Heightened sensitivity to light, sound and smell
- Elation or unusual energy

2. Aura

An aura is a clear neurological symptom. It occurs in 10% of migraine sufferers. It lasts from a few minutes to up to an hour. There may or may not be a gap between the end of the aura and the start of the headache phase. Features include:

- Visual disturbance
- Motor or sensory disturbance

3. Headache

During this phase, apart from the headache other associated features can occur:

- The headache is unilateral or shifting
- Phonophobia
- Photophobia
- Nausea
- Osmophobia (smell)
- Most are off their food, but some are extra hungry in spite of the nausea
- Often prefer to lie down in a dark room

4. Resolution and Recovery

- Lethargy and generally being "washed-out"
- Some have extra energy
- Can last up to a few days

Migraine triggers

In more than 50% of cases no trigger factor is apparent. The cause is often an accumulation of events rather than a single factor:

- Stress (emotional or physical) and anxiety
- Foods containing the amines, such as tyramine (cheese, chocolate, red wine)
- Bright lights
- Loud noise
- Exercise
- Hunger

Scenario

Ms. A had no preceding or family history of headaches/migraines. She describes the headaches as pounding and lasting most of the day. They occurred around the temple, usually left, but could occur on the right. Either way they progress to involve both sides. However whilst the headaches were moderately severe there were no other associated features such as nausea, vomiting, photophobia, osmophobia or phonophobia. She found stress could bring them on, but there were no prodromal symptoms or aura. She takes paracetamol, which eases the headaches. They occur once or twice a week.

Thus, at this point in time, the working diagnosis is still either tension-type headaches or migraine.

Examination

Blood pressure, pulse rate and fundoscopy help to exclude all those conditions associated with raised intra-cranial pressures and hypertension. Proper fundoscopy is not often performed in general practice due to the lack of completely dark rooms and/or dilating eye drops. However it should always be possible to see the optic disc and immediate surrounds (unless the patient has cataracts or corneal damage) and so the doctor should be able to visualise venous pulsation. That is, to see the veins emerging from the optic disc pulsating. The absence of this might be an early sign of raised intra-cranial pressure. Its presence thus helps to strongly exclude this possibility.

ENT and cervical spine examination takes minutes and must be done to exclude those possibilities. Cranial nerve examination is also essential in all headaches. I would suggest that the central nervous system is always examined for two reasons:

1. Patient reassurance that the doctor is taking the problem seriously (and is thus reassured)

2. Medico-legal

If temporal arteritis is a possibility, do not forget to palpate those arteries—they should be pulsatile and non tender.

Finally, the worst—a full neurological examination. Here is the good news! It takes less than 5 minutes to perform a full neurological examination in a family practice setting on a healthy subject. Here is how:

*   Get the patient to stand up (checks for muscle power, co-ordination plus understanding)
*   Get them to walk a few paces up and down (checks for cerebellar lesions and muscle power)
*   Ask them to walk with one foot immediately in front of the other (i.e. pigeon toed)
*   Ask them to walk on their toes and then on their heels (checks muscle power, long tract nerves, co-ordination and balance)
*   Ask them to stand with feet slightly apart. Close their eyes. Raise their arms to shoulder height with fingers spread apart. Tap their hands up or down (checks for Romberg's sign)

You can check reflexes if you want but if all the examination is normal and there is nothing sinister in the history, reflexes is likely to be normal. So really the full examination takes less than 5 minutes.

> ### Scenario
>
> In Ms. A's case the examination was all normal. All the sinister causes have been excluded by virtue of the history and normal examination. Cervical spine and ENT examinations were normal too. Thus the possible diagnoses remain the same.

Investigations

As is often the case, the less you do the better.

- FBC (anaemia has been known to cause headaches)
- ESR (only if temporal arteritis is a possibility)
- C-reactive protein (only if temporal arteritis is a possibility)

The use of plain X-rays (for sinusitis) has at best limited use. A plain lateral skull X-ray may well show enlarged pituitary fossa or calcification due to a tumour but is far from the best investigation for these problems. Similarly if sinusitis is a possibility invariably there is frontal and/or maxillary sinus tenderness. If ethmoidal sinusitis is a possibility then the type of headache would point to that, i.e. immediately behind the eyes, worse on bending forward, possible temperature and usually nasal symptoms. If you are that concerned then discussion with the neurologist or appropriate specialist would be a better option.

> ### Findings and results
>
> In this example, no investigations are warranted.

Management of headaches

Initial management

The diagnosis is still unclear, as sometimes does happen. There are distinct features of migraine but they are not conclusive. Sometimes patients can have both migraine and tension headache.

If it is thought that the cause is psychosomatic then the management is obviously to acknowledge and deal with the underlying cause, i.e. that the headache is due to the subconscious feeling of hurt or, to put it another way, the "head aches as it is feeling pain". Now this is often easier said than done, as many people do not wish to acknowledge that they have a mental health problem. In society, "being strong" means not showing emotions and dealing with all the insults that life can throw at you. But here is a thought … If we had a burst water pipe, how many of us could deal with it and not call a plumber? It is the same if the car engine goes wrong or indeed if we break a leg. So why should it be any different for our emotions? If we have a problem why is it not all right to ask for help? Put in this way, the patient is more likely to accept help and talk, especially if it is then said to them that in fact a "strong person" is the one who can admit that they cannot do everything for themselves and, at times, seeks help. It is "the weak" who are fearful of their feelings and store them up.

Thus if the cause is acknowledged, the problem is taken seriously and the doctor is seen to be empathetic, then many patients will acknowledge the possibility of the psychological aspect—it can then be put to them that by dealing with this aspect, the "pain" then goes and so will the headache. There are two options—either to refer to a neurologist and wait for the consultant's opinion or to try a pragmatic approach. Neither migraine nor tension headaches are life threatening. The aim is to try and identify which type of headache Ms. A has. It is possible that no matter how cooperative she is, she has not noticed any prodromal or precipitating features. Thus:

1. Ask the patient to keep a diary and to note the following:
a. When the headaches start (time and date)
b. How long they last
c. If there were any mood changes during the preceding 24 hours (check with friends or relatives to see if they have noticed any change)
d. When she had the headaches were there any other symptoms
e. What did she do to relieve the headaches
f. Were there any possible triggers, e.g. feeling stressed, certain sorts of food, related to menstruation, poor sleep, alcohol intake (and type)

2. Simple analgesics

Get Ms. A to take simple analgesics and to return with the diary after a period of time, say 4–6 weeks. As she is getting the headaches twice a week there should be enough data to try to define if there are other features of migraine.

Four–six week follow-up management

Ms. A returns with a fully completed diary. Unfortunately, as sometimes happens, it is not very rewarding from the point of view of confirming migraine. So what is next? Pragmatism!

Discuss the situation with Ms. A and ask what she would like to do. On the one hand she may be happy to know that there is nothing sinister, that it is possibly migraine but no more than that, and she finds she can cope by occasionally taking simple analgesics or even taking them prophylactically. Always make a proviso in these circumstances that she can return at any time if she becomes worried, if the headache changes in any way or if there are other new features. On the other hand, she may say that the headaches interfere too much with her life or that simple analgesics do not work or that she would like to know if this is migraine or not. In these circumstances, a trial of therapy is warranted.

In this case, two options are available. Again these must be discussed fully with the patient—let her make a joint decision as she has to take the drugs and be content with the decision.

Option 1

To try migraine relievers only, e.g. $5HT_1$ agonists also known as "Triptans" (e.g. sumatriptan, zolmitriptan). If taking these medications relieves the headache then it is reasonable to say she has migraine.

Option 2

If this is migraine, as the headaches are twice a week, it would be reasonable to consider prophylactic treatment. When to use prophylactic treatment is invariably up to the patient to decide. If the migraines were less than once a month not many people would want to take medication daily. If daily, almost all would. The options include pizotifen or a β-blocker (such as propranolol, metoprolol, nadolol or timolol). These are the most often used and recognised prophylactics each with their own contra-indications. Other possibilities include tri-cyclic antidepressants such as amitriptylline, sodium valproate and calcium antagonists, but none are licensed for this use.

Summary

At the end of this trial either the headaches have improved in some way (i.e. it is migraine) or they have remained the same. If the latter, the patient may wish to see a neurologist. This is not an unreasonable referral.

References

Migraine Action Association UK and "Simplified diagnostic criteria for migraine" (after Goadsby and Olesen [1996] and adapted from the International Headache Society), from http://www.migraine.org.uk/index.aspx.

van Gijin, J. and Rinkel, G. J. E. 2001. "Subarachnoid haemorrhage: Diagnosis, causes and management". *Brain*, 124(2): 249–278.

Chapter 16

Lower Back Pain

♦ Martin LINDSAY ♦

Scenario

A 65-year-old man comes in complaining of lower back pain for the last week or two.

What are the likely diagnoses and how do you proceed to make a final diagnosis?

The most likely causes

- Osteoarthritis/Spondylolisthesis
- Mechanical, i.e. muscular, ligamentous, facet joint dysfunction
- Prolapsed intervertebral disc (PID)

The important possibilities that (may) need to be excluded

- Cancer (primary or secondary)
- Infective, e.g. TB, osteomyelitis, discitis
- Inflammatory, e.g. ankylosing spondylitis, sacroilitis, Reiter's Syndrome, psoriatic arthropathy

The rare or unusual possibilities

- Radiated to back from elsewhere, e.g. abdomen, pelvic pathology (e.g. fibroids, endometriosis, pelvic infection if female, prostatitis if male)
- Spinal stenosis causing cauda equina compression

Symptoms are not unique

Pain and severity per se do not help in the establishment of the cause. What one person perceives as "mild" would be considered as "excruciating" by others. For example, a patient walks in complaining of severe lower back pain and promptly sits down. It is unlikely that their pain (if due to mechanical causes) is severe, as sitting would increase the pressure (and therefore the pain) in the lower back.

Similarly sciatica is due to pressure on the sciatic nerve—it gives no clue as to the cause of pressure, e.g. PID, cancer or inflammation due to infection or other inflammatory process.

Students should also be aware that in the majority of lower back pain cases, the cause is often not found. It is usually referred to as mechanical lower back pain in primary care, i.e. part muscular, part ligamentous, part posture related. Often it does not really matter, as the vast majority of lower back pains are self-limiting and resolve in spite of (or despite) doctors!

Symptoms pattern

A good history is crucial for distinguishing the simple causes of lower back pain from the more important causes such as those causing nerve root involvement or the sinister pathologies.

The importance of nerve root involvement is because the underlying cause may be a sinister pathology and/or if the pressure is not relieved, the nerve may be permanently damaged.

Specific questions to ask that may help

- The mode of onset at times can be most helpful. Was it following some form of trauma? Has the patient been doing some strenuous form of exercise in the preceding day or two? Is there a previous history of back problems?

- The classical way of getting a PID is to lean forward, rotate to the left or right, and then lift (a heavy) object. Thus the importance of asking the patient what they were doing at the time of onset of the pain.

Remember that a disc, in simple terms, is a "jelly encompassed by a mould". The net effect of the forward flexion is compression of the anterior part of the disc by the adjacent vertebrae. This causes minimal bulging of the disc anteriorly. On rotating, the anterior-lateral aspect of the disc is then pinched even more by the same vertebrae. At this critical point, the person then lifts a heavy object. For this to happen, the back muscles have to contract. The effect of this is to bring the two vertebral bodies closer together. The only thing preventing the two vertebral bodies from coming together is the disc. Thus the pressure inside the disc increases. In normal circumstances, i.e. the person is erect and upright, the vertebral bodies are kept apart at more or less their usual distance, as the compression effect is uniform throughout the disc. In this particular situation, however, the disc is already compromised as it is already in a compressed position. The pressure on the disc builds up not in a uniform way across the whole of the disc, but primarily in that same small area (anterior-lateral aspect). As the pressure continues to build, the jelly will eventually be squashed out and so creates a prolapsed disc.

How different causes present

Think about, in broad terms, the causes of lower back pain. By doing this, you can almost predict how the symptoms will present. For example:

Mechanical pain

Mechanical pain can be thought of as overstretched or bruised muscles and ligaments. Just like walking on a sprained ankle, the more you walk the worse the pain.

This is indeed what you find too for back pains. The patients complain their pain is worse with movement, and after prolonged standing or sitting. Why sitting? If you look at pressure in the lower back, the position causing the least pressure is lying supine. Lying on your side increases pressure slightly more whereas standing increases it a lot more. There is only one situation that is worse than sitting for increasing the pressure in one's lower back and that is sitting whilst leaning forward! (Back to those discs again!) Thus on sitting the damaged lower back muscles have to work overtime and so does the pain.

Beware not to be confused by the fact that there may also be associated tearing of fibres—not to the point of rupture or even partial rupture, but at a more microscopic level. In these circumstances there will also be an inflammatory healing process. Thus, on waking, the patient may be worse but find that their pain eases with gentle movements or as the day goes by.

The theory here is that, during the period of rest, the oedema (due to the healing inflammatory process) builds up. Use of the muscles then squeezes out this oedema so the patient feels better. Overuse of the muscle though will make the pain (and inflammation) that much worse (in simple terms if the ligament/muscle fibres are torn but healing, overuse will tear them again so making the pain worse again). So a bit of a mixed picture could well emerge.

For mechanical lower back pain, there may also be a previous history of the same.

Nerve root pain

If nerve roots are involved, e.g. PID then the pressure on the nerves will cause sharp electric shock type pain, paraesthesia, or numbness in the dermatomes supplied by the affected nerve. There may be muscle weakness too. If the nerve has been affected for some time there may also be associated muscle wasting

Pure inflammatory pain

We use the term "pure" to help you differentiate in your mind those true inflammatory causes such as ankylosing spondylitis and the other inflammatory arthropathies from those associated with a healing process (see mechanical pain above). As for above, these patients get morning stiffness that is eased by exercise and movement.

How to tell the difference between mechanical and pure inflammatory pain?

The history provides most of this information.

Where is the pain located? For example, all lumbar (ankylosing spondylitis), paravertebral (facet joint dysfunction), sacroiliac, etc., all give clues.

When was the onset? If ongoing for months, then it is "pure" inflammation. If after lifting and recent, it is likely to be mechanical.

How to tell if it is PID?

Does the pain radiate? It does that if there is nerve root involvement.

*   What is the patient doing to bring on the pain? It is usually an acute episode—invariably associated with forward flexing and rotating.

• Is the pain brought on by or made worse by coughing, sneezing, defecating, or on micturition?

Especially if there is a history of PID, anything that increases the intra abdominal pressure acutely can cause a PID. Why? To increase intra-abdominal pressure, all the muscles have to contract and these include the lower back muscles. If they do not contract then theoretically, contracting only the anterior abdominal muscles will push the abdominal cavity backwards! On contracting the lower back muscles, as explained above, there is increased pressure on the discs—if one or more of these discs have been weakened, then they will bulge.

Don't forget the rare causes

The history taking should also include other areas of the body if the history is not immediately compatible with the common causes, i.e. exclude abdominal, pelvic or cardiovascular problems. With men over 45 automatically include a prostate screen.

Classically the abdominal causes of back pain that radiate directly through to the back are:

• Aortic aneurysm or rupture
• Duodenal ulcer
• Pancreatitis

The conditions which radiate around the abdomen to the back are:

• Bilary colic, e.g. cholecysitis or cholelithiasis
• Renal colic

The sinister questions

The following list would suggest worrying features of back pain ("red flag" signs) and further elucidation may be required:

• Severe nocturnal pain
• Pain is worsening
• Pain not related to movement
• Isolated area of severe tenderness or pain
• Systemic symptoms or signs, e.g. weight loss, pyrexia, night sweats
• Incontinence of bowel or bladder
• Neurological features not limited to a single nerve root
• Neurological features that are progressive

- Back pain for the first time in young (< 20) or older patient (> 45)
- Thoracic pain is more sinister than lumbar pain

A working diagnosis

Scenario

A 65-year-old man comes in complaining of lower back pain. He gives a history of intermittent lower back pain for a few years. His last episode of back pain was 1 year ago. During that episode, his previous family doctor had arranged an X-ray of his back. It showed the presence of osteophytes suggestive of osteoarthritis. Currently the pain has been present for the last week or two. He has tried simple analgesics, which ease the pain. It is localised to the lower back. There is no weight loss or other sinister features. No genito-urinary or neurological symptoms. No other joint problems. He has had psoriasis since he was a young man. Ten years ago, he had a trans-urethral resection of prostate (TURP) for confirmed benign prostatic hypertrophy (on histology).

Thus at this point, the most likely possibilities are osteoarthritis (because of the evidence from his X-ray) and muscular pain. PID is not particularly likely to present for the first time in this age group unless there is a preceding history of the same.

Another possibility, however, is psoriatic arthropathy. Evidence against the latter is that there is no other joint involvement and that there was no sacroiliitis on examination. These usually accompany the condition. The previous family doctor made no mention to the patient of evidence of psoriasis on his X-ray, and he has only had back pains for the last few years.

Examination

The examination will determine the functioning of the back and legs. It includes noting the precise area of pain, how the back moves, power/ sensation in the legs, checking reflexes and straight leg raising.

Beware of those who say they cannot forward flex more than 20 or 30 degrees due to pain but can sit comfortably in a chair. They probably do have pain but not as severe as they are trying to make you believe (in both situations there is forward flexion of the spine). However if the patient comes in in a forward flexed position, is unable to forward flex any further due to pain, and when asked to sit down does so tentatively and usually only on the edge of the seat, then they do have a severe and genuine problem.

Here are some noteworthy examination pointers that might help

If the patient is able to forward flex to > 75 degrees, there is no need to perform straight leg raising (SLR) as this is going to be normal. It is said that if SLR is less than 30 degrees it probably is not a PID, and other causes need to be sought.

In PID, pain is worse on forward flexion compared to extension. It is increased further by forward flexing and swinging/rotating to the left or right (depending which side the prolapse is on).

For facet joint dysfunction and mechanical pains, the pain is worse on extension. To identify if this is facet joint or other mechanical, e.g. muscular, perform the Quadrant Test. This test or manoeuvre compresses the facet joint and so should increase the pain. It is performed as follows:

Get the patient to stand upright. Ask them to relax. Gently extend the back maximally. The patient's knees must not bend. Then laterally-flex and rotate the back towards the side of the pain.

The Slump Test is another useful test for sciatic nerve involvement. It is more sensitive than SLR. If there is sciatic nerve involvement the patient gets discomfort or a burning type sensation in their buttock or the back of their leg. If this happens they must bend the knee immediately. If the nerve is trapped, by performing this manoeuvre you have stretched the nerve. If not released it could lead to damage of the nerve.

To perform the test:

- Ask the patient to sit on the edge of the couch and literally slouch (It is probably a good idea to re-enforce the notion that they should never do this normally as bad posture like this causes back pain!)

- Place chin on chest
- Straightened the unaffected leg (they should have no discomfort)
- Straighten the affected leg. If no problems ask them to repeat but this time dorsiflex the foot too
- To differentiate between sciatic nerve and hamstring pain get the patient to lift their chin off their chest and repeat the leg raising. In sciatic nerve entrapment, the discomfort is then eased

Scenario

In this particular case, the gentleman's examination was not particularly remarkable. No particular points of severe tenderness. Movements in all directions were limited due to pain but not severely so.

Clinical Diagnosis

Thus psoriatic arthropathy is almost certainly excluded and osteoarthritis the most probable cause.

Investigations

In most cases of lower back pain, there is NO need to perform any investigations. However if the pain is prolonged, becoming worse, or there are other features in the history that make you suspicious, then it is reasonable to do so. Such investigations include:

- Full blood count (general screen to include leukaemias, etc.)
- ESR (for inflammatory arthropathies and malignancies)
- C-reactive protein (for inflammatory arthropathies and malignancies)
- Calcium/Alkaline phosphatase (raised in presence of bony metastases)
- Prostate specific antigen (screen for cancer of the prostate but can be raised with other prostatic conditions too, e.g. prostatitis and benign prostatic hypertrophy)
- Plain lumbar-sacral spine
  - ❖ Routine lumbar spine X-rays should be avoided as they invariably provide no useful information and make no difference to the management. The presence or absence of abnormality does not

confirm or refute pain. The presence of reduced lumbar lordosis can be found on careful examination and only means there is muscle spasm. This too should be discovered clinically. Further, there is no association between severity of osteoarthritic changes on the X-ray and the patient's symptoms. The presence of PID should be determined clinically because a reduced disc space is not always easy to determine on X-ray and if substantial would in any event be confirmed clinically.

❖ So when should it be done: If there is a suspicious history of sinister pathologies, e.g. cancers (even though plain X-rays only show metastases if there are associated sclerotic changes), infections, inflammatory disorders, or the pain is not easing after a reasonable period of time (especially in patients over the age of 45).

• Others—MRI
This is the definitive test. It will show the presence of tumours, inflammation and PID.

Scenario

For this gentleman, given his age, and the fact that the symptoms have been present for 2 weeks and that simple analgesics gave only partial relief, all the above blood tests were arranged, but not an X-ray as there was no specific tenderness in the spine and no weight loss.

Management of lower back pain

Initial management

General principles—most back pains are self limiting and so do not need much in the way of treatment. It is also well recognised that if someone has back pain, they soon learn which manoeuvres or activities bring on the pain. They then start to experience the pain before even doing those movements so promulgating their muscle spasm, pain and disability. To help prevent this vicious circle, it is essential to provide adequate analgesics and rapid mobility.

The general advice is as follows:

- Do not sit, except for eating and going to the toilet, as this maximises the pressure in the back
- Lie flat, stand or walk about
- If lying flat, place a pillow behind the knees and/or a rolled up towel in the small of the back (this makes lying more comfortable)
- Walk about and exercise as much as possible. Bed rest has no real part to play. Patients may be confined to bed for a few days due to their pain but this should not be considered as part of the treatment
- Try to gradually increase their physical activities over the subsequent days or weeks and encourage their return to work as soon as possible
- Adequate analgesics (see below)
- Physiotherapy or osteopathy if the problem is not resolved within a few weeks

Drug therapy

As already noted, adequate analgesics are essential not only for the obvious relief of pain but also to prevent possible chronic pain. Muscle spasm is an integral part of back pain. The trouble with this is that part of the continuing problem with back pains is that the tensed muscles do not relax and allow the spine to resume its normal position, thus prolonging any pain and healing process. Through relieving pain the muscle spasm can start to ease, thus allowing the spine to relax and so promoting resolution. So:

- Regular analgesia as required
- Use simple analgesics such as paracetamol with or without codeine. Non-steroidal anti-inflammatory drugs (NSAIDs), e.g. ibuprofen or diclofenac are very useful as adjuvants but be wary especially in the elderly due to incipient gastric bleeds
- Consider the short-term use of a muscle relaxant, e.g. baclofen, methocarbamol or diazepam

Nerve root pain

Family doctors, provided there is no progressive or major motor weakness, can initially manage nerve root pain in exactly the same way as above.

If the nerve root pain is not resolved within 4-6 weeks then the doctor should consider urgent referral to their local orthopaedics or rheumatology department.

If features of cauda equina syndrome are present then referral to orthopaedics/neurosurgery is required (urinary and faecal incontinence, sensory numbness of the buttocks and the backs of the thighs, lower motor neurone weakness, i.e. loss of dorsiflexion of the foot and toes, and of eversion and plantar flexion. The ankle jerks are usually absent on both sides).

Scenario

He was given the above advice and suitable analgesics and told to return 1 week later.

Findings and results

On returning he was more or less the same with no change to his symptoms. The results on this gentleman came back as all normal except his PSA was dramatically raised (suggestive of cancer). He was therefore urgently referred to the urologists.

Follow up

Results from the urologists confirmed prostatic cancer. Note that a TURP does not remove the entire prostate and especially the sub-capsular area where cancers first start.

His bone scan was normal. His back pain was due to osteoarthritis.

Summary

In summary, taking a good history and examining the patients properly are the most important steps in managing lower back pain. Family doctors should avoid over-investigation in these patients. Adequate analgesics are the first-line treatment of most patients but be mindful that many patients are not compliant as they worry about the side-effects and dependence. The aims are to keep them mobile and family doctors should consider physiotherapy or osteopathy if there is no improvement.

Chapter 17

Knee Pain

◆ Christopher TONG ◆

Scenario

Mr. Chan is a 28-year-old office worker who plays in his local football league. He injured his right knee 2 days ago during a football tackle and presents to his family doctor with knee pain. Two years ago he "sprained" the same knee, and ever since then he has noticed that his knee is "unstable" when playing certain sports.

What are the likely diagnoses and how do you proceed to make a final diagnosis?

The most likely causes

- Meniscus injury
- Anterior cruciate ligament injury
- Collateral ligament injury (medial or lateral)
- Posterior cruciate ligament injury

The important possibilities that (may) need to be excluded

- Fracture
- Cartilage injury (osteochondral injury) of the knee
- Injury to extensor mechanism (e.g. patellar tendon rupture)
- Tendonitis

Specific questions to ask that may help

The patient presents with knee pain after an injury, so the list of differential diagnoses pertains to traumatic knee conditions giving rise to pain.

The following questions (from history taking) will help differentiate the different differential diagnosis.

- *Site of the pain*
  The site of the pain is important. Ask the patient to point to where the pain is. If he localises the pain to the medial side of the knee, then possibilities are medial meniscus tear or medial collateral ligament tear. Similarly, this applies to the lateral side. Pain associated with cruciate ligament tears is less well defined. The patient may simply say the pain is "inside the knee". If the pain is in the front of the knee (patella/ patellar tendon) then injury to the extensor mechanism must be borne in mind.

- *Mechanism of injury*
  When the leg is "forced laterally" (i.e. a valgus force is applied), this is associated with a medial collateral ligament injury. When the leg is "forced medially" (i.e. a varus force is applied), this is associated with a lateral collateral ligament injury. When the foot is planted on the ground, and a twisting force is applied to the knee (pivoting force is applied), this is associated with an anterior cruciate ligament injury.

- *Swelling of the knee*
  Enquire whether the knee swelled up after the injury. And if it did, how soon after the injury did the swelling occur?
  Diffuse swelling of the knee after an injury is usually due to fluid accumulation within the knee. If this swelling occurs very soon (within a few hours) after the injury, it is likely due to blood in the knee (haemarthrosis). If the swelling comes on several hours after an injury (or swelling is noticed the day after injury), the swelling is likely due to an effusion rather than blood.

Causes of haemarthrosis after a knee injury
1. Anterior cruciate ligament tear
2. Fracture
3. Osteochondral injury (cartilage injury)
4. Peripheral meniscal tears

Causes of effusion after a knee injury
1. Meniscal tears
2. Collateral ligament tears

- *Presence of locking or reduced range of motion*
  After an acute knee injury, it is common to have reduced range of motion of the knee. This reduced range of motion may be due to true mechanical blockage, or just be secondary to pain and swelling within the knee. Common causes of true mechanical blockage would be a meniscal tear or a loose body. A loose body may be secondary to an osteochondral injury where a flap of cartilage is torn off and forms a loose body within the joint.

  We need to emphasise that after an acute knee injury, it is often difficult to differentiate between a true mechanical blockage and a reduced range of motion secondary to pain and swelling only. Repeat examination in a week's time (which is quite safe) when the pain and swelling is considerably reduced will help differentiate the two.

- *Feeling of giving way*
  In Mr. Chan's case, it is important to note from his history that he had a knee injury two years ago and that since then he had noticed his knee gives way, especially when he was playing contact sports or when he had to rapidly change direction when running (e.g. playing squash, tennis, etc.). This suggests that he may have sustained a ligament injury, e.g. anterior cruciate ligament injury two years ago, making the knee unstable and prone to further injury.

Further information gained from Mr. Chan after further history taking:

- Mr. Chan localised the pain over the medial side of the knee
- During the tackle he felt the leg being "swept outwards" (i.e. valgus force applied to knee) by his tackler
- He noticed swelling of the knee the day after the injury
- He could not fully extend the knee, but was unsure whether there was anything blocking movement
- Since his first knee injury two years ago, the knee often "gave way" or felt unstable when playing pivoting sports or contact sports

In Mr. Chan's case, he may have sustained a ligament injury two years ago making his knee unstable and prone to further injury. The medial side knee pain suggests a medial meniscus tear and/or medial collateral ligament injury. His inability to fully extend the knee may be due to a mechanical blockage. The swelling of the knee is likely an effusion rather than haemarthrosis, based on the speed on which it came on.

Examination

What to focus on in the physical examination of Mr. Chan's knee?

The examiner would use the physical examination to look particularly for a medial meniscus tear, medial collateral tear and anterior cruciate ligament tear. However all other structures should be examined as well.

Determine the presence of fluid swelling of the knee

Loss of medial knee dimple and a fullness of the suprapatellar pouch (as seen during inspection) also suggest fluid swelling in the knee. Small amount of fluid is best demonstrated by fluid displacement test. Large amounts of fluid collection are best demonstrated by patellar tap test.

Localise the exact site of tenderness

Accurate determination of exact site of tenderness is particularly helpful for diagnosing meniscal tears, collateral ligament tears and fracture.

Meniscal tears: Pain is localised to the joint line. Be sure to accurately localise the joint line.

Collateral ligament tears: Pain is often localised to either the femoral or tibial attachment of the medial collateral ligament. Medial collateral ligament tears are more common than lateral collateral ligament tears.

Bony tenderness may indicate fracture. Carefully palpate all bony landmarks.

Range of motion (ROM)

Determine any loss of range of motion, and whether there is a difference between active and passive range of motion. Ensure integrity of extensor mechanism by asking the patient to perform a straight leg raise.

Special tests

Perform special tests to determine integrity of the following structures (details of these tests can be obtained from physical examination textbooks):

- Anterior cruciate ligament: Lachman test and anterior drawer test
- Posterior cruciate ligament: posterior drawer test
- Medial collateral ligament: valgus stress test of the knee
- Lateral collateral ligament: varus stress test
- Menisci: Apley grinding and McMurray test

After an acute knee injury, complete physical examination may be difficult to conduct due to pain and swelling in the knee. Certain tests may be impossible to perform, e.g. McMurray test for meniscal tears as the patient needs to be able to fully flex the knee for the examiner to carry out the test.

Observations

There was gross swelling of the knee with positive patellar tap. Tenderness was localised to the medial joint line. There was no tenderness over the femoral and tibial attachment of the medial collateral ligament or on the lateral side of the joint. Femoral and tibial condyles were non tender. Range of motion was limited at 20 to 90 degrees only. He was able to perform straight leg raise. It was very difficult to perform any of the special tests due to the significant pain and swelling of the knee.

Conclusion after physical examination

The physical examination suggested that there was a medial meniscus tear (medial joint line tenderness) and that there may be a mechanical blockage within the joint (limited ROM). However little information was gained from the "special tests" as these were impossible to perform due to pain and swelling in the knee.

Investigations

*   *Knee X-ray*

    This will show the presence of any fractures and also any effusions though this should be found clinically

*   *Knee aspiration*

    Knee aspiration will show whether the fluid is blood or an effusion. Also knee pain may be considerably improved after aspiration of a tense effusion due to relief of pressure within the knee. However before embarking on knee aspiration, be sure to be trained in and familiar with the technique. Most importantly, knee aspiration MUST be done under aseptic technique to prevent iatrogenic infection.

Management of knee pain

1. *Ice*

    Apply ice to the knee. A practical approach is to get a bag of prepacked peas from the supermarket and put it in a freezer. Apply the bag of frozen peas to the knee 4 times per day for 15 minutes each time. Place a thin layer of cloth between the frozen peas and the skin to avoid cold injury to the skin. Icing the knee reduces pain, swelling and inflammation of the knee.

    Give the patient a tubigrip or compression bandage to reduce the swelling.

    Advise the patient to elevate the leg whilst at home.

2. *Explanation to patient*

    Explain to the patient the likely injured structures. Use a knee model to explain the anatomy (show them the meniscus and ligaments) or use an anatomy book. Explain to the patient that due to the swelling and effusion it is difficult to carry out a complete physical examination at the first clinic visit. Ask the patient to return to the clinic in one week's time for re-examination.

3. **Simple analgesics**

Prescribe paracetamol or an anti-inflammatory for pain relief.

Scenario

The patient returns to the clinic for follow up after one week. The findings show normal knee X-ray and no fracture. Patient reports that the knee pain is now much improved and the swelling has reduced considerably. He can fully extend the knee but still has pain when he fully flexes the knee (suggesting a meniscal tear).

Physical examination shows a positive fluid displacement test but negative patellar tap test (because amount of fluid in the knee has decreased). Medial joint line is tender on palpation. ROM 0–125 limited by pain (other knee ROM 0–130). This time able to carry out special tests: Lachman and anterior drawer tests positive suggesting anterior cruciate ligment tear. McMurray and Apley grinding tests resulted in pain localised to the medial joint line suggesting medial menisus tear. Valgus and varus stress tests negative suggesting intact collateral ligaments.

Working diagnosis

*   Anterior cruciate ligament tear
*   Medial meniscus tear

Investigations

MRI: Particularly good for looking for meniscal tears, cruciate ligament tears and collateral ligament tears. It can also pick up fracture and cartilage injuries.

Further management

A physiotherapist will be able to help the patient control the swelling of the knee and teach the patient exercises so as to help regain as much range of motion as possible. In addition the exercises taught by the physiotherapist help to prevent muscle wasting of the thigh muscles. After any kind of knee injury, muscle wasting can occur rather quickly and exercises to prevent this are important for early rehabilitation of the injured knee. These exercises include straight leg raises, semi-squats and cycling on an exercise bike.

The physiotherapist also plays an important role in educating the patient on the type of injury he has sustained, any precautions for future sporting activities and preventative measures for sustaining a further injury.

Referral to orthopaedic surgeon

If the patient has a locked knee and MRI confirms a meniscal tear, urgent referral to an orthopaedic surgeon is recommended, as any mechanical blockage inside the knee should be rectified as soon as possible.

On the other hand, if a patient has sustained a knee injury and there is swelling in the knee, but the patient can fully extend the knee (i.e. not a locked knee), then the doctor can review the patient in one week and assess progress. If there is no progress and the knee remains painful and swollen then referral to an orthopaedic surgeon is suggested. On the other hand, if the knee swelling is reducing, range of motion is improving and pain is getting better, then observation by the family doctor can be continued.

SECTION III

 ✑

Problem-based Diagnoses and Management in the Specific Groups

Chapter 18

Acne Vulgaris

◆ Antonio CHUH ◆

> ### Scenario
>
> Ms. M is a non-smoker and non-drinker. She is sexually inactive. Past health is good. She has regular 28–30 days menstrual cycles. Drug history is unremarkable. She has no history of illicit drug use.
>
> Examination reveals greasy face. Open comedones (blackheads) and closed comedones (whiteheads) are seen with inflammatory papules. Papules and pustules are seen. Cysts and abscesses are not evident. Early coalescence of lesions is seen. The angles of the jaws are affected. Depressed scars are present. No keloid is seen.
>
> Her trunk, shoulders and upper arms are spared of lesions. No evidence of hirsutism is noted. She is not obese.

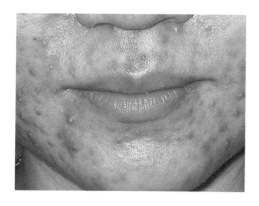

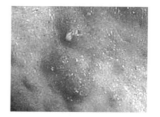

What are the likely diagnoses and how do you proceed to make a final diagnosis?

The most likely cause

- Acne vulgaris

The important possibilities that (may) need to be excluded

- Perioral dermatitis
- Allergic contact dermatitis
- Irritant contact dermatitis
- Rosacea
- Drug-induced acne (combined oral contraceptive pills, phenytoin, barbiturates)
- Polycystic ovarian syndrome

The rare or unusual possibility

- Virilising tumours

Symptoms are not unique

Acne vulgaris is not the only possible cause of papular lesions on the face. The application of topical corticosteroids may lead to perioral dermatitis. However comedones are not seen in this dermatosis. The application of topical remedies including the topical antibiotic might lead to allergic or irritant contact dermatitis. The age of Ms. M and the presence of open and closed comedone render rosacea less likely. However facial erythema, telangiectasia, and papules/pustules particularly affecting the forehead, cheeks and chins should be looked out for.

Acne might be primary or secondary. Drug-induced acne is probably the commonest cause of secondary acne.

Owing to the history of regular menstrual cycles and the absence of hirsutism on examination, causes of virilisation including polycystic ovarian syndrome need not be considered at the present moment. Such possibilities should be reconsidered should her lesions remain recalcitrant despite active intervention.

Acne can present with inflammatory and non-inflammatory lesions. Both are now present on the face of Ms. M. Her acne is moderately severe at present. There is no evidence of acne conglobata (coalescing nodulocystic acne with abscesses) or acne fulminans (severe cystic acne with suppuration of lesions, fever and polyarthralgia). The effect of the lesions on her psychosocial well-being is eminent. The major complication of acne is scarring.

There exists convincing evidence that acne is associated with significant psychological morbidities including depression, anxiety and numerous psychosomatic symptoms (Tan 2004). Social morbidities include embarrassment and social inhibition (Tan 2004). There is local data (Chuh and Chan 2005) and plenty of data worldwide supporting the view that the quality of life of patients with acne is significantly affected.

The psychosocial effect, i.e. the singularity of acne is likely to be particularly pertinent for adolescent patients, as they are in a stage of developing self-identity (Smith 2001). Physical appearance is important for their self-image and confidence.

Symptoms pattern

Many women notice that the severity of their acne changes according to their menstrual cycle. Many patients also notice that certain types of food such as greasy food or chocolates may precipitate acne. However there exists no convincing evidence that food is significantly associated with acne, and no evidence that food avoidance is beneficial for the prevention, control and treatment of acne. The same applies to personal hygiene.

Smoking has been shown to be a significant risk factor for acne vulgaris in males but not females (Chuh et al. 2004).

Many patients notice worsening of acne during periods of emotional stress such as before examinations. Thus it is worthwhile exploring with the patient any known or perceived associations that cause the acne to worsen.

Specific questions to ask that may help

- Severity of symptoms, e.g. pain
- Effects on her self-image, e.g. loss of self-confidence
- Effects on her mood, e.g. depression, lack of sense of self-worth, loneliness
- Effects on her daily activities, e.g. work, shopping, choice of clothes, application of makeup, isolation

- Effects on her interpersonal relationships, e.g. friends, colleagues
- Effects of her treatments, e.g. adverse reaction, financial burden

Grading

The Leeds Acne Grading System (Burke and Cunliffe 1984) is an established tool in assessing severity in acne vulgaris. It is applied by visual comparison of the severity of a patient's inflammatory lesions against a standard panel of photographs. One panel suitable for use in primary care consists of 16 photographs, with eight showing facial lesions, four showing chest lesions and four showing back lesions. The grades range from 1 (very mild) to 12 (exceptionally severe).

A working diagnosis

The diagnosis is highly likely to be acne vulgaris of moderate severity, without evidence of secondary organic cause.

Examination

Hiadradenitis suppurativa sometimes accompanies severe acne. Inflammatory nodules, abscesses, hypertrophic scars and keloids can be looked for in the axillae and anogenital regions if there is a history of intermittent pain and inflammation in those areas. Otherwise, further examination might not be necessary at this point unless a differential diagnosis or a secondary cause of acne is suspected.

Scenario

Acne vulgaris, moderate severity with evidence of scarring, no evidence of secondary organic cause.

Investigations

Investigations to search for androgen excess are unnecessary at this point unless signs of virilisation or hirsutism are evident. Investigations may then include early morning cortisol, free testosterone, sex hormone binding globulin, follicle stimulating hormone, luteinising hormone, and ultrasonography of the ovaries and adrenal glands.

Liver function tests, fasting cholesterol and triglycerides, fasting glucose and pregnancy test may be necessary before commencing oral retinoid therapy. Such tests fall largely within the remit of the dermatologist.

Management of acne

Initial management

As already discussed, there exists adequate evidence that effective treatment of acne exerts significant beneficial impacts on the self-esteem and confidence of patients (Tan 2004). Encouragement and support from the family doctor combined with appropriate intervention should be offered. Myths such as the roles of hygiene and diet should be actively dispelled. If the patient is male it may be more appropriate to also discuss the adverse effects of smoking on acne.

Family doctors should be prepared to discuss the pros and cons of the treatment options with patient. The patient should then make an informed decision as to whether they would like to have active intervention. The modality of treatment most suitable is governed by the severity of the disease and the psychosocial impacts perceived by the patient.

Adolescent patients should be encouraged to get involved in the decision-making process. Aspects to consider include not only physical and psychological ones but also the financial burden of treatment on the family. For patients with severe nodulocystic acne or significant scarring on presentation, the need of referral to a dermatologist should be discussed.

Acne vulgaris with mild severity can be managed with topical therapy, usually in the form of topical antibiotics including clindamycin or erythromycin, benzoyl peroxide gel, topical retinoids, or topical azelaic acid. In general, topical antibiotics are more effective for inflammatory lesions (pustules and papules) while topical retinoids are more effective for non-inflammatory lesions (closed and open comedones).

Benzoyl peroxide

Benzoyl peroxide is available over the counter as cream, gel and wash preparations. Its action in acne vulgaris stems from its antibacterial properties. Effects may not become obvious until 4–6 weeks after commencement of therapy. There is also a variable degree of drying and peeling effect, which may help to prevent a relapse.

Adverse effects include erythema, peeling and irritant contact dermatitis. About 3% of individuals are truly allergic to benzoyl peroxide and an allergic contact dermatitis may develop (Shwereb and Lowenstein 2004). It may bleach hair or fabric.

Combination products of benzoyl peroxide and topical antibiotics may prevent the development of antibiotic resistance and confer improvements in patients who have already developed resistance (Taylor and Shalita 2004).

Topical antibiotics

Ms. M confirmed that she had been [softer and sounds more polite] applying the clindamycin solution spot-by-spot. She noticed no improvement in her lesions. The absence of symptomatic remission is likely to be related to her using the wrong method of applying the solution. Topical antibiotics exert their anti-comedogenic activity by decreasing the colonisation of propionibacterium acnes. They should thus be applied to the entire face. Application is usually twice daily.

Adverse effects of topical antibiotics include skin dryness, irritation, peeling and dermatitis. Patients truly allergic to the antibiotic might develop allergic contact dermatitis. Antibiotic-related pseudomembranous colitis is theoretically possible with topical clindamycin, but such cases are very rare.

Topical retinoids

Topical tretinoin and isotretinoin have an anti-comedogenic effect and promote peeling of affected skin areas. They may also be useful against solar-aging and for wrinkles. Application is usually once daily or once every 2–3 days. Lesions may worsen initially before improvement is seen in 2–3 weeks. Adverse reactions include burning, stinging, pigmentation, depigmentation and dermatitis. They also increase the chance of photosensitisation and the use of sunscreens may be recommended. For this reason application is advised at night.

While the conventional topical retinoids are mainly used for non-inflammatory acne, newer retinoids such as adapelene and tazarotene have anti-inflammatory effects (Millikan 2003). Their roles in acne treatment in primary care remain to be demonstrated.

Azelaic acid

Azelaic acid has antibacterial effects which may be attributable to inhibition of bacterial protein synthesis. At high concentrations it is bactericidal against propionibacterium acnes (Charnock et al. 2004). It is effective for acne vulgaris of mild to moderate severity. Application is usually twice daily. Effects may not be appreciated in the initial four weeks of treatment. Adverse effects include dryness of skin, burning, stinging and dermatitis.

Some patients like azelaic acid owing to its effect of lightening hyperpigmented skin, and the skin is not usually lightened to beyond normal skin complexion. For this reason azelaic acid is sometimes prescribed to patients with melasma.

Follow-up management

A trial of topical treatment should be maintained for at least two to three months. If no remission is evident, systemic treatments might be considered.

Systemic treatment by the family doctor is usually in the form of oral antibiotics or hormonal therapy.

Systemic antibiotics

Systemic antibiotics can be prescribed alone or added to topical antibiotics. The usual ones are oral tetracycline 1–2 g daily, oral doxycycline 100 mg daily or oral erythromycin 1–2 g daily. Ms. M should be advised that the course of treatment will last for at least 4–6 months. Treatment response might be seen as early as two weeks, but might be delayed for up to 6–8 weeks after commencement of therapy.

Oral tetracycline should be taken with an empty stomach. Its absorption is also impaired by milk and antacids. The absorption of oral doxycycline is also impaired by antacids, although to a lesser extent than for tetracycline. Both tetracycline and doxycycline are contraindicated in pregnancy. Tetracycline is usually twice to four times a day, whilst doxycycline is once a day. For both these reasons doxycycline is often preferred although it is more expensive. Oral minocycline is likely to be effective in acne vulgaris. However many types of minocycline-induced irreversible hyperpigmentation have been described (Mouton et al. 2004), the uncertainties regarding its safety profile render it inappropriate as a first-line treatment (Garner et al. 2003).

Oral erythromycin not unusually causes gastrointestinal adverse reactions such as abdominal cramps and diarrhoea. Its use is usually considered when a course of doxycycline fails, or if the patient is sensitive to tetracyclines.

The roles of other antibiotics such as roxithromycin in acne vulgaris are also being explored (Ferahbas et al. 2004).

Hormonal therapy

The usual treatment is cyclical packs of tablets with cyproterone acetate 2 mg and ethinylestradiol 0.035 mg. The first pack should be started on the first day of menstruation. One tablet is taken daily for 21 days, followed by a tablet-free period of seven days before commencement of another pack. It is no more effective than oral antibiotics.

Adverse reactions include nausea, abdominal distension, breast distension, increase in body weight, intermenstrual bleeding, melasma and depression. Contraindications include pre-existing pregnancy, lactation, liver diseases, thromboembolic states, focal migraine, hypertension and oestrogen dependent tumours. The patient should be warned that although such a preparation has contraceptive effects, there exists a risk of contraceptive failure as per all combined oral contraceptive pills.

There is evidence that several combined oral contraceptive pills have beneficial effects on acne. However how their efficacies compare with each other and with other treatment modalities for acne is yet unknown (Arowojolu et al. 2004). Some combined oral contraceptive pills (e.g. Microgynon 30) are relatively androgenic and as such can worsen acne.

Indications for referral

A referral to a dermatologist should be considered if the lesions are not responding to treatment, if new lesions keep on erupting despite active treatment, or if acne keloids are present. If Ms. M is very concerned about her lesions and her appearance then discussions about a dermatological referral can take place.

Systemic retinoid

Among other treatments, the dermatologist might consider systemic isotretinoin for Ms. M. This is the only medication which causes histological changes to the pilosebaceous units leading to remission of acne vulgaris. Treatment is usually for four to six months. Relapse is still possible but the chance of relapse is much lower than for other modalities of treatment.

Systemic isotretinoin is highly teratogenic. Affected infants have face asymmetry, thymus aplasia and congenital heart defects. Ms. M must adopt reliable contraceptive methods during the months on therapy, and continue such methods for at least one month after cessation of therapy. The use of barrier contraception alone is not a reliable contraceptive method.

Adverse effects include dryness of skin, dermatitis, exfoliative chelitis, transient alopecia, myalgia, arthralgia, changes in the liver enzymes, hypertriglyceridaemia, hypercholesterolaemia, and effects on the eyes and musculoskeletal system (Charakida et al. 2004).

The association of systemic isotretinoin therapy with anxiety, depression and suicidal thoughts is still controversial (Hull and D'Arcy 2003; Ferahbas et al. 2004). Such risks have to be balanced against the risk of depression associated with acne itself (Hull and D'Arcy 2003). Patients should be fully counselled of the pros and cons by the dermatologist before decisions on treatment are made.

Management of scars

Ms. M should be advised that picking the papules will leave scars. A Cochrane review concluded that it is controversial whether laser resurfacing is effective for facial acne scars (Jordan et al. 2001). However camouflage cosmetics is an effective alternative.

References

Arowojolu, A., Gallo, M., Grimes, D. and Garner, S. E. 2004. "Combined oral contraceptive pills for treatment of acne". *Cochrane Database of Systematic Review*, 3: CD004425.

Burke, B. M. and Cunliffe, W. J. 1984. "The assessment of acne vulgaris—The Leeds technique". *British Journal of Dermatology*, 111: 83–92.

Charakida, A., Mouser, P. E. and Chu, A. C. 2004. "Safety and side effects of the acne drug, oral isotretinoin". *Expert Opinion on Drug Safety*, 3: 119–129.

Charnock, C., Brudeli, B. and Klaveness, J. 2004. "Evaluation of the antibacterial efficacy of diesters of azelaic acid". *European Journal of Pharmaceutical Sciences*, 21: 589–596.

Chuh, A. T., Zawar, V., Wong, W. C. W. and Lee, A. 2004. "The association of smoking and acne in men in Hong Kong and in India—A retrospective case control study in primary care setting". *Clinical and Experimental Dermatology*, 29: 597–599.

Chuh, A. A. T. and Chan, H. H. L. 2005. "The effect on quality of life in patients with pityriasis rosea—Is it associated with rash severity?" *International Journal of Dermatology*, 44: 372–377.

Ferahbas, A., Turan, M. T., Esel, E., Utas, S., Kutlugun, C. and Kilic, C. G. 2004. "A pilot study evaluating anxiety and depressive scores in acne patients treated with isotretinoin". *Journal of Dermatological Treatment*, 15: 153–157.

Ferahbas, A., Utas, S., Aykol, D., Borlu, M. and Uksal, U. 2004. "Clinical evaluation of roxithromycin: A double-blind, placebo-controlled and crossover trial in patients with acne vulgaris". *Journal of Dermatology*. 31: 6–9.

Garner, S. E., Eady, E. A., Popescu, C., Newton, J. and Li, W. A. 2003. "Minocycline for acne vulgaris: Efficacy and safety". *Cochrane Database of Systematic Review*, 1: CD002086.

Hull, P. R. and D'Arcy, C., 2003. "Isotretinoin use and subsequent depression and suicide: Presenting the evidence". *American Journal of Clinical Dermatology*, 4: 493–505.

Jordan, R. E., Cummins, C. L., Burls A. J. and Seukeran, D. C. 2001. "Laser resurfacing for facial acne scars". *Cochrane Database of Systematic Review*, 1: CD001866.

Millikan, L. E. 2003. "The rationale for using a topical retinoid for inflammatory acne". *American Journal of Clinical Dermatology*, 4: 75–80.

Mouton, R. W., Jordaan, H. F. and Schneider, J. W. 2004. "A new type of minocycline-induced cutaneous hyperpigmentation". *Clinical and Experimental Dermatology*, 29: 8–14.

Shwereb, C. and Lowenstein, E. J. 2004. "Delayed type hypersensitivity to benzoyl peroxide". *Journal of Drugs Dermatology*, 3: 197–199.

Smith, J. A. 2001. "The impact of skin disease on the quality of life of adolescents". *Adolescent Medicine*, 12: 343–353.

Tan, J. K. 2004. "Psychosocial impact of acne vulgaris: Evaluating the evidence". *Skin Therapy Letter*, 9: 1–3, 9.

Taylor, G. A. and Shalita, A. R. 2004. "Benzoyl peroxide-based combination therapies for acne vulgaris: A comparative review". *American Journal of Clinical Dermatology*, 5: 261–265.

Further reading

Berson, D. S., Chalker, D. K., Harper, J. C., Leyden, J. J., Shalita, A. R. and Webster, G. F. 2003. "Current concepts in the treatment of acne: Report from a clinical roundtable". *Cutis*, 72 (1 Supp.): 5–13.

Leyden, J. J. 2003. "A review of the use of combination therapies for the treatment of acne vulgaris". *Journal of American Academy Dermatology*, 49 (3 Supp.): S200–210.

Lo, K. K., Chong, L. Y., Tang, Y. M. W. and Ho, K. M. *The Handbook of Dermatology and Venereology.* Social Hygiene Service, Department of Health.

Useful websites

AcneNet: www.skincarephysicians.com/acnenet/
Acne support group: www.stopspots.org/
American Academy of Dermatology: www.aad.org/pamphlets/acnepamp.html
British Association of Dermatologists: www.bad.org.uk/public/leaflets/acne.asp
NHS Direct: www.prodigy.nhs.uk/guidance.asp?gt=Acne%20vulgaris

Patient information leaflets

DoctorUpdate: www.doctorupdate.net/du_toolkit/du_patientleaflets.asp
JB Medical: www.jbmedical.com/pil-acne.htm
Postgraduate Medicine: www.postgradmed.com/issues/2002/11_02/pn_acne.htm

Chapter 19

Atopic Dermatitis

◆ Antonio CHUH ◆

Scenario

J is a 6-year-old boy who has had generalised itchy skin rash since the age of eight months. He keeps on scratching during the daytime and at night. Sleep is disturbed. J also has frequent episodic asthma and allergic rhinitis. His father had asthma as a child and his mother had "eczema" in childhood.

J is now given baths with diluted emulsifying ointment twice daily in the winter, and once daily in summer. His mother is very concerned about long-term adverse effects of topical corticosteroids, and thus is reluctant to apply such medications prescribed for J. J is on budesonide inhalation 200 µg once daily via a spacer device, with terbutaline inhalation also via aerochamber on a "when required" basis. He is on occasional courses of fluticasone nasal spray for two to three weeks when his rhinitis symptoms are severe.

J's mother has previously requested a private laboratory to perform a radioallergosorbent assay (RAST) for J. IgE against housedust mite and a fairly wide range of food was reported to be elevated. J was consequently not given milk, dairy products, eggs, beef and any seafood. However no symptomatic improvement of his skin condition was noted on such restrictive diet.

Examination revealed dry skin with erythematous lesions on trunk and flexor aspects of four extremities. Excoriations are evident, but crusting and lichenification are minimal.

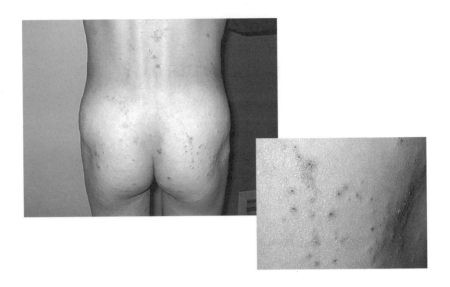

What are the likely diagnoses and how do you proceed to make a final diagnosis?

The most likely cause

- Atopic dermatitis (atopic eczema)
  These two terms are synonymous. In the United Kingdom, eczema tends to mean idiopathic whereas secondary causes result in dermatitis. In the USA all are referred to as dermatitis.

The important possibilities that (may) need to be excluded

- Secondary infections, e.g. virus (herpes simplex, molluscum contagiosum, viral warts), bacteria (impetiginisation by staphylococci and streptococci) and fungi (dermatophytes and candida)
- Scabies
- Ichthyosis vulgaris

The rare or unusual possibility

- Hyperimmunoglobulin E syndrome (hyper IgE syndrome)

Symptoms are not unique

The early onset of symptoms before the age of one and the chronic nature of the dermatosis are highly suggestive of atopic dermatitis. The presence of other atopic conditions and positive family history further support the diagnosis.

The diagnostic criteria proposed by the United Kingdom Working Party (Williams et al. 1994) are fulfilled. A simplified version of the criteria is as follows.

To diagnose atopic dermatitis the patient must, during the last year, have suffered from: a condition of itchy dermatitis (perhaps reported by the parents). This is an essential sign.

Associated are three or more of the following signs:

1. A history of skin lesions affecting the (insides of the) elbows, the popliteus, the ankles, the sides of the neck (including the cheeks in children under ten)
2. A personal history of asthma or allergic rhinitis (or a history of atopic illness in first degree relatives in children under four)
3. A history of dry skin over the past year
4. Eczema visible when flexed (or in children under four localised on the cheeks/forehead and/or the outside of the limbs) at the time of examination
5. Onset before the age of two (not valid for children under the age of four)

Secondary bacterial and viral infections are common and should be under constant review. Sensitive clinical signs of impetiginisation include weeping, crusting, periauricular fissures and small pustules (Lubbe 2003). Eczema herpeticum and eczema molluscatum are the commonest secondary viral infections in atopic dermatitis (Wollenberg et al. 2003). Viral warts are sometimes seen. Scabies is possible but unlikely unless there exists a contact history (household members developing generalised itch recently or their cat/dog developing an itchy rash) or suggestive signs such as burrows or penile papules.

Ichthyosis vulgaris (autosomal dominant ichthyosis) might mimic atopic dermatitis (Tay et al. 2002). Family history of dry itchy skin can be present in both. Other atopic manifestations such as asthma and allergic rhinitis are common in both conditions. A fish-scale pattern should be looked for, particularly on the shins. Keratosis pilaris is usually marked.

Palmoplantar creases are accentuated. Note that the axillae, antecubital fossae and popliteal fossae are usually spared in ichthyosis vulgaris. The face can be affected in early childhood but face involvement is unusual for older children and adolescents. Other types of ichthyosis are usually severe enough to cause little diagnostic confusion with atopic dermatitis.

Various congenital syndromes including Wiskott-Aldrich syndrome and hyper IgE syndrome have a pronounced atopic element. They should be considered if the dermatitis is exceptionally severe and recalcitrant to therapy. Gluten-sensitive enteropathy is rare in Chinese.

Hyper IgE syndrome is probably underdiagnosed as the immunocompromising element can be variable and thus a typical history of recurrent pyogenic infections may not be volunteered unless specifically asked for (Hsu et al. 2004). The inheritance, although being autosomal dominant in most circumstances, has high variability of penetrance and thus absence of family history does not exclude the disorder. Fortunately in the case of J, RAST has been performed and although total IgE is elevated it is not in the region of thousands which would be expected for hyper IgE syndrome.

Symptoms pattern

Scratching is an aggravating factor. Secondary bacterial (staphylococcal, streptococcal) and viral (herpes simplex viruses, pox virus, human papillomavirus) infections might precipitate widespread dermatitis. Cold dry weather might exacerbate atopic dermatitis. The role of food is often emphasised by the parents, but food avoidance usually has little role in the clinical management. Emotional factors are of relevance, particularly for older children, adolescents and adults.

Specific questions to ask that may help

- Severity of symptoms, e.g. itch
- Effects on his self image, e.g. loss of self confidence
- Effects on his mood, e.g. unhappiness
- Effects on his daily activities, e.g. schooling, choice of clothes
- Effects on his leisure activities, e.g. difficulties when entering swimming pools, changing rooms, the beach

- Effects on his interpersonal relationship, e.g. friends calling him names
- Effects on his sleep
- Effects of his treatments, e.g. time-consuming to apply and washing of garments due to the grease, his mother's concerns about side-effects of topical corticosteroids, sedation effect of oral medications

Grading

The SCORing Atopic Dermatitis (SCORAD) index (European Task Force on Atopic Dermatitis 1993) is an established tool in assessing severity in atopic dermatitis. The index assesses atopic dermatitis by extent, severity and subjective symptoms. The extent of the rash is marked on two diagrams showing the anterior and posterior trunk and limbs of the patient. The percentage of body surface area involved is then estimated. Severity is assessed by six parameters: redness, swelling or roughness, oozing or crusting, scratch marks, thickening of skin and deeper skin crease (lichenification), and dryness of unaffected skin. Each parameter is assessed on a scale of 1–3. Subjective symptoms are assessed by two parameters of pruritus and sleep loss, each on a visual analogue scale of 1–10. The individual scores are entered into a programme for a final score to be computed.

SCORAD itself is too tedious to be applicable to daily management for children and adults with atopic dermatitis in primary care. However the components of the index are of genuine relevance in assessing the severity of atopic dermatitis. The family doctor should remember that he is assessing three aspects: the area of involvement, the manifestations in six parameters and the subjective symptoms.

Of direct relevance to management is the impact of atopic dermatitis on the quality of life of J. This can be objectively assessed using the Children Dermatology Life Quality Index (Lewis-Jones and Finlay 1995), a validated Cantonese version of which is available (Chuh 2003).

A working diagnosis

The diagnosis is highly likely to be atopic dermatitis.

Examination

Further examination at this point should aim at evaluating for signs of secondary bacterial infection, viral infection and ectoparasitic infestation. Common accompanying conditions, including ichthyosis vulgaris, juvenile plantar dermatosis, keratosis pilaris and pityriasis alba, should be examined for. Should pityriasis alba be suspected, examination under Wood's light might help in distinguishing such from pityriasis versicolor.

Clinical diagnosis

Atopic dermatitis, asthma, allergic rhinitis.

Investigations

Further investigations are not likely to be necessary at this point. If impetiginisation is suspected, treatment can be commenced but skin swabs for bacterial culture adds little to the treatment decisions except if there is no initial response. For widespread vesiculations, Tzanck smear or vesicular swabs for herpes virus DNA by polymerase chain reaction might be considered, although clinical diagnosis might suffice in most circumstances. Clinical diagnosis is also usually adequate for molluscum contagiosum.

If scabies is suspected skin scraping for microscopy is indicated, not only to document the infestation but also to assure compliance as the whole family and not J alone should be put on scabicidal treatment.

RAST and prick tests to document type I hypersensitivity have little role in the care for a child with atopic dermatitis in primary care. Their injudicious use might lead to over-emphasis on diet manipulation, as has occurred in the case of J.

Management of atopic dermatitis

Initial management

Time spent in counselling J and his parents is time worth spent. Their concerns, expectations, level of acceptance and knowledge of this chronic condition should be appreciated. Otherwise the parents might keep on taking J on doctor-shopping tours, or continue looking for miracle cures.

J and his parents should be reassured that although there is no permanent cure for atopic dermatitis, good control is often possible.

Avoidance of allergens and irritants

Avoidance of allergens is already being carried out by J's parents in the form of diet restrictions. Such restriction based on the results of a single RAST test results might not be beneficial for J in the long-term. Whether these restrictions might be so strict as to cause nutritional deficiencies is also an issue of concern and so should preferably be under the supervision of a dietitian.

Cross-reactivity is common for RAST tests, and interpretation is always difficult. If J's parents have genuine concerns, it may be wise to refer J to an allergist or a paediatric dietitian rather than to continue a restrictive diet with no proven benefit. The implication of possible cow's milk protein intolerance should be discussed in detail with the allergist. Oral food challenge remains the gold standard in the diagnosis of food allergy (Perry et al. 2004).

That IgE against housedust mite is highly positive is expected for most children with atopy. It has been demonstrated that measures of housedust mite avoidance exert significant impact on the severity of atopic dermatitis (Tan et al. 1996). Mattresses and pillows can be encased. The top covers can be cleaned regularly by washing in at least 60°C water. In the case of daily clothing, woollen and synthetic fibres are irritants. Cotton and silk are better (Ricci et al. 2004).

Emollients

The use of emollients should be continued. This is the mainstay of treatment. J is already on diluted emulsifying ointment for his baths. Creams and lotions can also be advised, to be applied all over the body twice daily in winter and once daily in summer. In cooler and dryer climates emollient may need to be applied even more frequently. However J's parents should be discouraged from purchasing excessively expensive proprietary preparations which might not have additional benefits but may add to the already heavy financial burden of atopic dermatitis on the family (Verboom et al. 2002).

If the atopic dermatitis is mild, aqueous cream may be applied as an emollient three or four times daily as needed to keep the skin greased and also as a soap substitute. Soap should not be used as it degreases the skin, the exception being for washing the hands for hygienic purposes. Sweat, being water soluble, is removed by ordinary washing with water.

If the atopic dermatitis is more severe, emulsifying ointment may be used as a soap substitute instead. Some patients also prefer to use emulsifying ointment directly on the skin.

Wet medicated dressings

During an acute flare-up, the family doctor can demonstrate to the family the use of wet medicated dressings. Although such dressings are usually applicable to hospitalised patients, home-based application for several days is possible if the parents are motivated enough and if they are properly taught the technique and given the necessary support (Bridgman 1994).

A water-based emollient is first applied all over the body. A topical corticosteroid cream is then applied to the areas with active dermatitis. The parents should be informed that redness and active itch rather than dryness are the keys to identifying such areas. A layer of wet dressing is then applied, followed by a double layer of tubular elasticated bandage. The dressings are changed two to three times daily for 3–5 days.

Follow-up management

Topical corticosteroids

Parents are likely to be apprehensive about the adverse effects of topical corticosteroids as widely covered in the press. They may also confuse the effects of topical corticosteroids with their systemic counterparts. Rather than over-application of such medications being a concern as was the case some 10–20 years ago, under-application of topical corticosteroids is now common for children with atopic dermatitis. J's parents should be informed that emollients are the mainstay of treatment and that topical corticosteroids are to be applied on an "as required" basis. They should be reassured that the strength, area, frequency and duration of application of topical corticosteroids prescribed are tailored to the individual child. Such application under appropriate medical supervision should be safe.

As for the choice of topical corticosteroids, a local study demonstrated that the use of "soft" steroids such as 1% hydrocortisone, 0.1% mometasone furoate and 0.005% fluticasone proprionate are effective in the treatment of atopic dermatitis, with the efficacy further improved by wet wraps (Pei et al. 2001).

Systemic antihistamines

If sleep is disturbed, sedating antihistamines can be prescribed as a single nocturnal dose. Contrary to traditional belief, there is some evidence that chlorpheniramine may not be effective in relieving pruritus (Munday et al. 2002). The newer non-sedating antihistamines are conventionally perceived as less effective in the control of pruritus which is not purely histamine-mediated as in the case of atopic dermatitis. However newer agents such as cetirizine have been reported to have no adverse effects on the behaviour or learning processes in young children with atopic dermatitis (Stevenson et al. 2002). Their efficacies warrant further investigations. The choice for the optimal systemic antihistamines is thus still controversial. In the United Kingdom, children are usually prescribed promethazine since brompheniramine is no longer available.

Topical immunosuppressive agents

Topical immunosuppressive agents including tacrolimus and pimecrolimus inhibit calcineurin and suppress T lymphocytic responses. They are effective for children with atopic dermatitis, and do not seem to cause skin atrophy. These agents may exert steroid-sparing effects in the design of a treatment plan for J. Apart from atopic dermatitis, these medications have been found to be useful in other types of dermatitis and autoimmune dermatological diseases (Chuh 2004b). However they are more expensive than topical hydrocortisone.

Pimecrolimus may be less potent in relieving pruritus than betamethasone valerate, while tacrolimus is as equally potent as betamethasone valerate (Williams 2002). A burning sensation may be experienced upon application of tacrolimus. This is not usually found for pimecrolimus. Results from further clinical studies, and the financial situation of the family, should be factors when considering the role of such medications in long-term management for J.

Leukotriene antagonists

Several clinical studies have reported the value of montelukast in treating atopic dermatitis (Rackal and Vender 2004). The value of leukotriene antagonists in the management of this condition remains to be shown.

Treatments to be considered by the dermatologist

There exists adequate evidence for the efficacy of ultraviolet phototherapy and systemic immunosuppressive agents such as cyclosporin in the treatment of atopic dermatitis in adults (Hoare et al. 2000). The roles of these treatments in children are controversial. The role of systemic corticosteroids in treating children with very severe atopic dermatitis is also controversial.

Alternative treatments

A systematic review failed to provide adequate evidence to recommend the use of Chinese herbs, homeopathy, massage therapy, hypnotherapy or evening primrose oil in the treatment of atopic dermatitis (Hoare et al. 2000).

Management of complications and accompanying conditions

Impetiginisation

If impetiginisation is likely, a course of topical fusidic acid ointment may be adequate if the condition is confined. The role of topical antibacterial-corticosteroid combination preparations is still controversial. Small areas of impetiginisation might be treated with such combination therapy (Williams 2000). However if larger areas are involved, appropriate doses of systemic antibiotics, e.g. flucloxacillin, or erythromycin if allergic to penicillins, might be indicated.

Eczema herpeticum and eczema molluscatum

Systemic acyclovir is the usual treatment for eczema herpeticum (Lai et al. 1999). J should be referred to a dermatologist if the diagnosis is uncertain or if the area of involvement is large. Eczema molluscatum can be troublesome. However it is not a dangerous condition (Wollenberg et al. 2003), and conservative treatment (observing for spontaneous remission) should be considered for the child.

Pityriasis alba

Pityriasis alba has been reported to be present in 25% of school children with atopic dermatitis (Tay et al. 2002). Treatment is usually conservative (observing for spontaneous remission) after pityriasis versicolor is excluded by proper examination under Wood's light. Skin scraping for the characteristic "meatball and spaghetti" appearance of pityrosporum orbiculare (malassezia furfur as hyphal form) under direct microscopy is helpful, but fungal culture is not.

Asthma and allergic rhinitis

These conditions should be under good control. A holistic management plan for J should cater for all his atopic conditions.

Juvenile plantar dermatosis

Juvenile plantar dermatosis frequently coexists with atopic dermatitis. A local study has reported that the quality of life of children with such condition is usually affected only to a limited extent (Chuh 2004a). Conservative management with proper shoe wear, protection against friction and emollients should suffice for most children. Acute exacerbations might necessitate the use of topical corticosteroids.

Keratosis pilaris

Keratosis pilaris is reported to be present in 13% of school children with atopic dermatitis (Tay et al. 2002). Treatment is conservative (topical emollients).

Ichthyosis vulgaris

Ichthyosis vulgaris is sometimes misdiagnosed as atopic dermatitis. It is reported to be present in 8% of children with atopic dermatitis (Tay et al. 2002). Treatment is mainly by emollients.

Summary

Patients with atopic dermatitis and their family members should be informed that atopic dermatitis is a chronic disease. There exists no permanent cure. However whether the condition is under good control or not exerts significant impacts on the quality of life of the patients and their families.

Avoidance of allergens is sometimes initiated by patients or their carers. Diet restriction is also a common practice. These approaches usually do not exert very appreciable impacts on the quality of life of the patients. Where necessary, allergen identification by investigations such as RAST might be considered, provided that the patients understand the limitations while interpreting the investigation results.

The importance of liberal application of emollients cannot be over-emphasised. Potent and acceptable preparations need not be expensive. While patients are experiencing an acute exacerbation, the application of emollients might paradoxically lead to more pruritus initially. Such reaction should be made known to the patients.

Topical corticosteroids might now be under-prescribed instead of over-prescribed in some geographic locations, as adverse effects of topical corticosteroids are usually known to patients and their families. Patients might also confuse the adverse effect of topical and systemic corticosteroid treatments.

Topical corticosteroid preparations should be prescribed at the appropriate strength, with the appropriate vehicle, at appropriate frequency of application, in appropriate durations, to the appropriate body parts, and with appropriate amounts prescribed or dispensed. Soft corticosteroids are also available with less local side-effects. However their prescription has to be balanced with the financial status of patients. Lectures and courses are available to pharmacists so that they might also be equipped with the correct attitudes, knowledge and skills in dispensing topical corticosteroids as well as counselling patients on the benefits and adverse effects of such medications (Chuh 2006–2008). Systemic histamine antagonists have a role in controlling the pruritus. Part of the antipruritic effects is related to their sedating effects. Thus older generations of sedative antihistamine preparations are useful and can be prescribed as a single noctural dose.

The indications and adverse effects of topical immunosuppressive agents are still controversial. Local and international guidelines should be referred to.

Complications of atopic dermatitis are common and should be actively anticipated, prevented and properly managed. Many children and adult patients with atopic dermatitis are also enduring concomitant atopic conditions, such as asthma, allergic rhinitis, allergic conjunctivitis and atopic urticaria.

References

Bridgman, A. 1994. "Management of atopic eczema in the community". *Health Visit*, 67: 226–227.

Chuh, A. A. T. 2006–2008. "Recognition and assessment of common skin problems in community care settings". The University of Sunderland, United Kingdom and School of Professional and Continuing Education, The University of Hong Kong.

———. 2004a. "Quality of life in children with juvenile plantar dermatosis in primary care settings". November 2004, Melbourne. 6th Australian Conference on Quality of Life. Hosted by the Australian Centre on Quality of Life.

———. 2004b. "The application of topical tacrolimus in vesicular pemphigoid". *British Journal of Dermatology*, 150: 622–623.

———. 2003. "Validation of a Cantonese version of the Children's Dermatology Life Quality Index". *Pediatric Dermatology*, 20: 479–481.

European Task Force on Atopic Dermatitis. 1993. "Severity scoring of atopic dermatitis: The SCORAD index". *Dermatology*, 186: 23–31.

Hoare, C., Li, W. P. A. and Williams, H. 2000. "Systematic review of treatments for atopic eczema". *Health Technology Assess*, 4: 1–191.

Hsu, C. T., Lin, Y. T., Yang, Y. H. and Chiang, B. L. 2004. "The hyperimmunoglobulin E syndrome". *Journal of Microbiology, Immunology and Infection*, 37: 121–123.

Lai, Y. C., Shyur, S. D. and Fu, J. L. 1999. "Eczema herpeticum in children with atopic dermatitis". *Acta Paediatr Taiwan*, 40: 325–329.

Lewis-Jones, M. S. and Finlay, A. Y. 1995. "The Children's Dermatology Life Quality Index (CDLQI): Initial validation and practical use". *British Journal of Dermatology*, 132: 942–949.

Lubbe, J. 2003. "Secondary infections in patients with atopic dermatitis". *American Journal of Clinical Dermatology*, 4: 641–654.

Munday, J., Bloomfield, R., Goldman, M., Robey, H., Kitowska, G. J., Gwiezdziski, Z., Wankiewicz, A., Marks, R., Protas-Drozd, F. and Mikaszewska, M. 2002. "Chlorpheniramine is no more effective than placebo in relieving the symptoms of childhood atopic dermatitis with a nocturnal itching and scratching component". *Dermatology*, 205: 40–45.

Pei, A. Y., Chan, H. H. and Ho, K. M. 2001. "The effectiveness of wet wrap dressings using 0.1% mometasone furoate and 0.005% fluticasone proprionate ointments in the treatment of moderate to severe atopic dermatitis in children". *Pediatric Dermatology*, 18: 343–348.

Perry, T. T., Matsui, E. C., Kay Conover-Walker, M. and Wood, R. A. 2004. "The relationship of allergen-specific IgE levels and oral food challenge outcome". *Journal of Allergy and Clinical Immunology*, 114: 144–149.

Rackal, J. M. and Vender, R. B. 2004. "The treatment of atopic dermatitis and other dermatoses with leukotriene antagonist". *Skin Therapy Letter*, 9: 1–5.

Ricci, G., Patrizi, A., Bendandi, B., Menna, G., Varotti, E. and Masi, M. 2004. "Clinical effectiveness of a silk fabric in the treatment of atopic dermatitis". *British Journal of Dermatology*, 150: 127–131.

Stevenson, J., Cornah, D., Evrard, P., Vanderheyden, V., Billard, C., Bax, M. and Van Hout, A. 2002. ETAC Study Group. "Long-term evaluation of the impact of the h1-receptor antagonist cetirizine on the behavioral, cognitive, and psychomotor development of very young children with atopic dermatitis". *Pediatric Research*, 52: 251–257.

Tan, B. B., Weald, D., Strickland, I. and Friedmann, P. S. 1996. "Double-blind controlled trial of effect of housedust-mite allergen avoidance on atopic dermatitis". *Lancet*, 347: 15–18.

Tay, Y. K., Kong, K. H., Khoo, L., Goh, C. L. and Giam, Y. C. 2002. "The prevalence and descriptive epidemiology of atopic dermatitis in Singapore school children". *British Journal of Dermatology*, 146: 101–106.

Verboom, P., Hakkaart-Van, L., Sturkenboom, M., De Zeeuw, R., Menke, H. and Rutten, F. 2002. "The cost of atopic dermatitis in the Netherlands: An international comparison". *British Journal of Dermatology*, 147: 716–724.

Williams, H. 2002. "New treatments for atopic dermatitis". *British Medical Journal*, 324: 1533–1534.

Williams, H. C., Burney, P. G., Pembroke, A. C. and Hay, R. J. 1994. "The UK working party's diagnostic criteria for atopic dermatitis. III. Independent hospital validation". *British Journal of Dermatology*, 131: 406–416.

Williams, R. E. 2000. "The antibacterial-corticosteroid combination. What is its role in atopic dermatitis?" *American Journal of Clinical Dermatology*, 1: 211–215.

Wollenberg, A., Wetzel, S., Burgdorf, W. H. and Haas, J. 2003. "Viral infections in atopic dermatitis: Pathogenic aspects and clinical management". *Journal of Allergy Clinical Immunology*, 112: 667–674.

Further reading

Barnetson, R. S. and Rogers, M. 2002. "Childhood atopic eczema". *British Medical Journal*, 324: 1376–1379.

Lo, K. K., Chong, L. Y., Tang, Y. M. W. and Ho, K. M. *The Handbook of Dermatology and Venereology.* Social Hygiene Service, Department of Health.

Useful websites

EczemaNet: www.skincarephysicians.com/eczemanet/index.html
National Eczema Society: www.eczema.org/
Skin Care Campaign: www.skincarecampaign.org/

Patient information leaflets

British Association of Dermatologists: www.bad.org.uk/patients/disease/atopic/
     atopic.asp
DoctorUpdate: www.doctorupdate.net/du_toolkit/du_patientleaflets.asp

Chapter 20

Hoarseness

◆ Stephen K. S. FOO, William P. T. YIP ◆

Hoarseness is a very common symptom that can affect anyone from the very young to the very old. Most people experience it after a long day of talking or indeed after going to a pop concert or sports event! However the term hoarseness can be used by the patients to describe a variety of vocal symptoms. It usually refers to a coarse or scratchy sound, often associated with a habitual clearing of the throat in an attempt to restore voice quality. Patients may refer to a feeling of dryness, tightness or choking in the throat.

Scenario

A 30-year-old female kindergarten teacher presents with a persistent dryness of the throat, cough and hoarseness for 3 weeks. As a member of a church choir she has difficulty singing high notes, which she used to be able to do. She has been treated with the usual antibiotics, cough mixtures and steam inhalations. Her cough and sore throat have improved but hoarseness persists.

What are the likely diagnoses and how do you proceed to make a final diagnosis?

The most likely causes

- Vocal abuse leading to laryngitis
- Vocal cord polyp formation (Singer's nodules)

- Reinke's oedema
- Non resolving upper respiratory tract infection causing post nasal drip

The important possibilities that (may) need to be excluded

- TB laryngitis
- Leukoplakia or neoplasm of the vocal cords
- Recurrent nerve palsy
- Gastroesophageal reflux laryngitis
- Psychogenic hoarseness

The rare or unusual possibility

- Cord palsy. However this is most unlikely as it would cause aphonia and bovine type of cough

Symptoms pattern

- Sudden onset of hoarseness or loss of voice is a rare event in the absence of trauma. Sustained bellowing and screaming can traumatise the vocal cords, which is the usual reason for this problem
- Traumatic life events can lead to psychogenic hoarseness and a careful history may help to establish this causal link
- A rapidly developing hoarseness typically occurs with acute inflammatory conditions such as allergic or infectious laryngitis
- Intermittent hoarseness can be linked to patterns of voice use or environmental factors, e.g. smoke. Thus occupational and social history must be carefully explored
- Chronic hoarseness is usually the result of chronic inflammatory disorder of the larynx. Thus a smoking history of marijuana and hashish as well as cigarette smoking history is important
- Reinke's oedema is another common but benign condition. Both vocal cords have an inflammatory and oedematous polypoidal appearance. It is due to severe vocal abuse and chronic irritation
- Physiological hoarseness: For example, a 10-year-old boy is observed having hoarseness for 2 weeks after the school sports day. He has no sore throat or other symptoms and is otherwise perfectly healthy. The likely diagnosis is non-specific laryngitis or vocal cord polyp. Another

likely condition is that the young boy is passing through the physiological voice breaking stage experienced by teenagers

- Chronic neurological disorders can affect the voice but again, it is uncommon for this symptom to occur on its own

- Cancer of the larynx is not common in the age group of this scenario. However in the over 50s a low threshold for including this should be included, especially if they smoke. It most commonly arises from the surface epithelium of the vocal cords but it may go unnoticed until airway obstruction or obvious voice change occurs.

Specific questions to ask that may help

- Laryngeal nerve paralysis can occur after surgery to the neck, thyroid or chest

- Spasmodic hoarseness is a condition which primarily affects women and is commonly mistaken for psychogenic hoarseness in that the voice is either strained, strangled or very weak

A working diagnosis

Scenario

A 50-year-old solicitor has been quite concerned about his health. He is a non-smoker and works out and plays tennis twice a week. He is happy that he shed 5 lb in the last month. A week ago he had a cold and went to see a herbalist. Instead of getting better, he woke up the next morning with bouts of coughing and lost his voice. He immediately went to consult his family doctor. He was treated for acute laryngitis with antibiotics. Seeing no improvement after 2 weeks, he requested a referral to an ENT specialist. Indirect laryngoscopy confirmed left vocal cord paralysis.

Examination

Before examining the larynx, attention should be given to the ears, nose, throat and neck, looking for signs of infectious or allergic sinonasal conditions or cervical masses (especially non-tender significantly sized lymph nodes). Simple vocal tasks help to evaluate the essential laryngeal functions of breathing, coughing, swallowing and phonation (e.g. sing up and down the scale). Full general ENT examination is not usually done by family doctors, but our ENT colleagues will conduct examinations such as indirect laryngoscopy (either with conventional mirror or endoscopes) to detect vocal cord mobility, polyps or other abnormalities of the vocal cords. In young children examination of the larynx is difficult. For our 10-year-old boy, if the cause is physiological, this is usually evident and voice abuse tends to settle after 1 or 2 weeks. Singer's nodules is rare in this age group as it is caused by chronic abuse. If the problem has not settled after 3 weeks he may need to be referred to an ENT specialist for an indirect laryngoscopy (with fibre-optic laryngoscope) under local anaesthetic (10% lignocaine) spray. Failing that an examination under general anaesthesia may be necessary. Before proceeding, the family doctor can consider a chest X-ray to exclude TB.

Investigations

Investigation is to establish the underlying cause of certain findings from history and examination such as recurrent nerve palsy. The point to note is that 30% of cord palsy is idiopathic and can recover spontaneously after a few months. Usually we wait for about 3 months before deciding on surgical medialisation of the cord. While waiting, we can recommend that the patient have speech therapy using the "pushing" technique to improve the quality of his voice and to allay his anxiety a bit. Another point to note is that even a healthy non-smoker can have carcinoma of the lung. Routine chest X-ray is a must in the investigation in the case of unilateral vocal cord immobility. Clinically ALL persisting hoarseness should have a chest X-ray to exclude TB, lung cancer or rarer lung conditions. Routine chest X-ray will also help to detect any pulmonary infection. Severe cases of reflux can be confirmed with oesophageal endoscopy.

 Congenital webbing or laryngomalacia is rare. The incidence of carcinoma is not that common except in industrial areas. With increasing age, the human voice deepens to a noticeable hoarseness level. In some such cases endoscopic laryngoscopy reveals tensor weakness of the vocal cord. Further investigations including videostroboscopy are quite academic and will not help in the treatment. There is no specific medication for this condition. Speech therapy can be of help if the symptom is disturbing.

The majority of cases of hoarseness are due to benign laryngitis or a polyp caused by vocal abuse. A thorough understanding of the patient's occupation and social activity and habits is of the utmost importance. In urban conurbations the hectic lifestyle, the noisy, polluted environment and the non-stop use of mobile phones inevitably have an undesirable effect on the vocal cords.

Management of hoarseness

There are certain circumstances that require more urgent attention or referral. They are:

- Long-standing history with recent stridor—this can be carcinoma

- Aphonia of recent onset or associated with neck surgery—cord palsy has to be ruled out

- Sudden stridor in children—this can be acute epiglotittis or a foreign body in the throat. This is an emergency. Send the patient to hospital or to a specialist immediately and NEVER use a tongue depressor because of the risk of causing laryngeal spasm and thus asphyxiation

If no obvious vocal lesions are identified on indirect laryngoscopy, general principles of vocal hygiene can apply:

- Vocal rest is difficult to achieve, so frequent breaks in talking should be scheduled throughout the day. Teachers or public speakers should be encouraged to use voice amplification devices

- Hydration with an increase of water intake and inspiration of vaporized water or saline is comforting. Lozenges and throat gargles are soothing but are of little benefit to the inflamed vocal cord lesions

- Anti-reflux measures in gastroesophageal reflux include avoidance of spicy food and alcohol, and head elevation. Consider the use of PPIs, compound alginate preparations and dopamine antagonists that promote gastric emptying such as metoclopramide/domperidone

- Quit smoking

Since voice disorders are often multifactorial (e.g. allergic or infective sino-laryngitis), treatments aimed at the underlying disorders are essential. Topical analgesics should be avoided as they encourage forceful phonation.

Most patients with voice disorders may benefit from the expertise of a speech therapist. Voice therapy is particularly useful in acquiring efficient phonation behaviour and preventing further vocal trauma. Psychotherapeutic intervention combined with an antidepressant may be helpful for some patients.

Hoarseness in professional singers is an entirely different category. The voice is an essential asset to their livelihood. They are extremely sensitive to the slightest change. All professional singers are well trained in how to use their voice and are very careful to protect it. Occasionally they do suffer from polyp or leukoplakia or even carcinoma. Slight dysphonia occurring just before the first day of a concert is common. It is the result of tension build-up and is a functional disorder that requires effective reassurance and symptomatic therapy. If the use of the voice is required in the immediate future, prompt referral to an otorhinolaryngologist may be necessary, when a systemic steroid may be prescribed.

 Summary

All in all, hoarseness must not be regarded as just another medical pathology. It is a broad functional and social disability which confronts family doctors probably more frequently than otorhinolaryngologists. A family doctor often sees patients coming into his practice fairly hoarse but complaining about something else. When asked about their voice, they often say the hoarseness has been present for a long time and does not bother them at all. An alert physician should explore their family background and occupation, and the significance of the hoarseness.

Not all hoarseness requires immediate indirect or direct laryngoscopy. If breathing is not affected and the patient is not a professional voice user, it is justifiable to assume infection and/or rhinitis as the cause and to treat the patient with the appropriate medication and advice on vocal hygiene as above. If there is no improvement in a week or two the patient should be referred for a chest X-ray and/or to an otorhinolaryngologist for further investigation.

Chapter 21

Acute Red Eye

◆ Donald LI ◆

The red eye is one of the most common ocular problems presenting to family doctors (estimated to be 40 per 1,000 consultations) and it can occur in all age groups. As a family doctor, we need to distinguish a few sight threatening conditions including acute glaucoma, iritis and keratitis, and scleritis/episcleritis, and make an urgent referral.

Scenario

Ms. L is a 35-year-old office executive in finance. Since yesterday evening, she noticed redness and discomfort of both of her eyes. Initially she thought her eyes were tired and this morning there was some sticky discharge. She did not wear prescriptive eyeglasses nor contact lenses. She was not on any medication and rarely saw her family doctor.

What are the likely diagnoses and how do you proceed to make a final diagnosis?

The most likely causes

- Infective conjunctivitis (about 75% of the cases)
- Subconjunctival haemorrhage
- Local irritation and affliction
- Allergy
- Blepharitis/Blepharoconjunctivitis

The important possibilities that (may) need to be excluded

- Glaucoma
- Corneal ulcer due to herpes trauma or foreign body
- Acute iritis

The rare or unusual possibilities

- Episcleritis
- Scleritis
- In association with other conditions, e.g. Reiter's Syndrome, ankylosing spondylitis, sarcoidosis
- Malingering

Symptoms are usually few

- One eye that is red, with or without discharge
- Both eyes are red, with or without discharge
- Red eyes that also happen to be painful
- Painful eyes that happen to be red

Symptoms pattern

Usually insidious onset with the patient noticing it when looking in the mirror or told by others. Sometimes may experience a gritty sensation or itchiness in the eyes that leads the patient to rub the eyes. Another scenario might be that the patient first notices discharge and then realises the eyes are red. Slightly unusually the patient may feel painful eyes and notice they are red.

Specific questions to ask that may help

- The three MOST important symptoms that help to exclude serious disorders of the anterior eye chamber and the cornea are:

  1. Painful eye: It is important to differentiate pain, itchiness or feeling of a foreign body. Severity of the pain also matters as acute glaucoma presents with severe pain, nausea and vomiting.

2. Any visual disturbance? Has the vision changed or reduced?

3. Does the bright light enhance the discomfort? (keratitis)

4. Any halos around bright lights? (acute glaucoma due to swelling and distortion of the cornea)

- When did Ms. L notice the red eye?
  Was one of the eyes red first? To establish whether it is acute, chronic or recurrent in nature, and any possible infectivity

- Any recent mood disturbance? (e.g. red eyes can be due to crying)

- History of
  - ❖ Wearing contact lens (keratitis is common in contact lens users)
  - ❖ Using cosmetics—eyeliners/mascara
  - ❖ Using eye drops

- Does she have a history of allergies and atopy?

- Any joint pain or non-specific aches and pains (as in connective tissue disorder, Reiter's Syndrome, ankylosing spondylitis)?
  Any history of high blood pressure?

- Is there a family history of connective tissue diseases?

- Nature of work—computer monitors and screens? (arc weldering)

- Always ask the patient what their concerns are—you cannot reassure anyone until you know for certain what is bothering them

A working diagnosis

In this case infective conjunctivitis is the most likely, although serious conditions such as glaucoma and iritis may need to be excluded by examination.

Examination

The eyes

Systematic inspection is the most powerful diagnostic tool for a family doctor in diagnosing acute red eye. Simple examination can be very revealing:

- Where is the redness: Whole sclera (e.g. scleritis—with pain and sometimes blurred vision) or only section (segmental, suggestive of haemorrhages or circular, suggestive of infective origin) of sclera? Superficial or deep (episcleritis vs. scleritis where the former involves the dilatation of episcleral capillaries and no pain)? Unless a family doctor has a split lamp, it is almost impossible to distinguish between scleritis/episcleritis (clue from history—in episcleritis the patient may have pain although usually far less than in the case of scleritis)

- Discharge—clear (allergic, especially if bilateral) or purulent (infective)?

- Any nodular lesion (episcleritis)? But this may not be obvious without the use of a split lamp, which is seldomly available in the family doctor setting.

- Pupil reflex—in acute glaucoma, the pupil is half dilated and fixed. In acute iritis, the pupil is spastic (small)

- Tenderness on palpation/Eye pressure—in acute iritis, the iris sphincter is irritated by the inflammation which causes pain. In glaucoma, the eyeball feels hard like a stone. In infants, check for the possibility of blocked lacrimal ducts by applying pressure over lower medial aspect corner of eye and check for improved drainage.

- Fluorescein stain and inspect the cornea looking for damaged corneal epithelium with a green light (keratitis/trauma)

- Do not forget to evert the eyelids to exclude foreign bodies

Dangerous symptoms are reduced vision, ocular pain and photophobia while dangerous signs include protusion of the eye, clouding of the cornea, abnormal pupils and pericorneal redness. These require immediate referral.

General

Fever? Any skin rashes/lesions? Posture (ankylosing spondylosis)?

If connective tissue related, other abnormalities may appear

Joint deformities and tenderness (e.g. sacroid or ankylosing spondylosis is associated with iritis).

Cardiovascular

Raised blood pressure; murmurs (rarely).

Clinical diagnosis

Apart from bilateral red eyes with a little yellowish discharge, all other findings were negative. The most likely diagnosis is infective conjunctivitis in Ms. L's case.

Investigations

Blood tests (very rarely indicated)

- Complete blood count (unlikely to be abnormal even in bacterial conjunctivitis)
- ESR, rheumatoid factor, C-reactive protein, connective tissue disease markers (if connective tissue disorder suspected)
- Urea and electrolytes (only if hypertension on history or examination)

Other investigations

- Tonometry—simple to use device and is available for family doctors. Fluorescein dye—the green dye will outline and stain defects when examined by torchlight—easy-to-use test strips are available
- Eye swab for culture and sensitivity—rarely necessary. May be considered for recurrent cases. The exception is ophthalmia neonatorum, i.e. conjunctivitis within a few days of birth, in which case perform an eye swab for microscopy, culture and sensitivity as well as for chlamydia.
- Split-lamp—probably better left to specialist

Findings and results

Final diagnosis is conjunctivitis, likely to be bacterial (see Table 21.1). Agree that it is infective conjunctivitis but the commonest cause is now said to be viral (just like urti/om—also that in children if urti and conjunctivits are present, then it is almost certainly viral and that even if bacterial the majority of cases can be settled without antibiotics). See www.clinicalevidence.com regarding antibodies vs. placebo.

Table 21.1 Comparing the clinical presentations of bacterial and viral conjunctivitis

Clinical Presentation	Bacterial Conjunctivitis	Viral conjunctivitis
Discharge	Purulent	Serous
Eye lids stuck together	Common	Uncommon
URTI symptoms	Rare	Common
Tearing	Moderate	Profuse
Number of eyes affected	One	Two
Palpebral conjunctiva	Papillae	Follicles
Preauricular adenopathy	Uncommon	Common

Management of red eye

The following approaches can be adopted:

- Avoid covering or irritating the eye. Natural history is for the condition to abate within a period of a few days

- When in doubt, it is safe to dilate a constricted pupil and constrict a dilated pupil by applying Gutt atropine (dilater) and Gutt pilocarpine (constrictor)

- Immediate referral to an eye specialist is mandatory in cases of suspected iritis or suspected penetration by foreign bodies or other serious eye diseases. Delay may lead to loss of vision

- Never take the risk of applying topical steroids when the diagnosis is in doubt. In the presence of dendritic ulcers, applying steroids amounts to malpractice. I would go even further and say that family doctors should never perscribe topical steroids unless directed and supervised by an ophthalmologist in confirming diagnosis and follow up to ensure there are no complications from the use of steroids

- The only treatment needed for spontaneous subconjunctival haemorrhage is explanation and reassurance (and to check their BP)

Initial management

- Treat and provide early relief for threatening serious conditions—should be referred immediately to eye casualty for conditions such as suspected glaucoma and acute iritis by pupil constrictors/dilators
- Arrange referral for serious eye injury cases
- Initiate antibiotic eye drops for suspected infection—traditionally chloremphenical eye drops (initially every two hours and then four times daily) and ointments have been the first line drug of choice. Availability of quinolones such as ciprofloxacin is a good alternative, or gentamycin. Fuscidic acid though available is not a logical choice as the majority of bacterial infections are due to streptococcus and a minimum due to staphylococcus.
- Review 3 days later if redness persists

Advanced management

- When a patient presents with recurrent infective conjunctivitis, family doctors should consider the possibility of chronic irritation due to atopy (and therefore itchiness) or secondary infection from frequent habitual eye rubbing. Screening for diabetes mellitus and other conditions associated with decreased immunity should also be considered
- Hand washing before handling contact lenses prevents contamination and possibly infection. Proper sterilisation and washing of contact lenses according to instructions using the appropriate solutions is important
- There is little evidence and support the view that health supplements benefit the eye except Vitamin A. The benefit of Chinese herbs such as *gou qi zi* (枸杞子, wolfberry) and natural foods such as bilberry needs verification. Proper daily cleansing of eyes is important to prevent accumulation of oil clogging the pores and causing irritation and inflammation of the eyelid, which promotes infection. If an individual has oily skin, they can consider gently scrubbing the pores with a piece of gauze soaked with diluted baby shampoo to remove any excess oily deposits. Before cleaning, remember to wash the hands

Chapter 22

"I can't do it, doctor!" (Erectile Dysfunction)

◆ William C. W. WONG ◆

Erectile dysfunction (ED) is common. The Massachusetts Male Aging Study of 1,709 men aged 40–70 years in Boston between 1987–1989 reported a prevalence of 52%. In Asia however geographical differences in prevalence exist[1-3], with a prevalence of ED ranging from 30% in Singapore to 78% in the Philippines[3]. With the aging population, ED is an important public health problem for men. However the social stigma related to this problem means that delay in seeking help, or simply ignoring the problem, is common. It is therefore very important that when a patient raises this issue, the doctor must demonstrate willingness to discuss it and address it with a good understanding of the topic. A patient-centred approach should be adopted to find out what has prompted this patient to choose to discuss it at this particular moment.

Erection involves the integration of neural and vascular functions and three neural mechanisms (psychogenic, reflexogenic and centrally originated, i.e. nocturnal erection) trigger the vascular changes required. Since 95% of spinal cord injury patients are capable of reflexogenic erections, 25% of patients with lower motor neuron lesions are capable of psychogenic erections and more than 90% of incomplete lesions of either kind retain their erectile function, the clinical presentation is often a mixed picture and sometimes even misleading.

Traditionally, most cases of erectile dysfunction were thought to be psychologically based, but it is now understood that most have an organic cause (80%), especially in older patients. In about 40% of men over 50, the primary cause is related to atherosclerotic disease. The role of smoking is controversial but it may amplify other risk factors such as hypertension or coronary heart disease. The mechanism of action in systemic diseases such as diabetes is often multifactorial. Therefore, in this case, we need to exclude chronic diseases and iatrogenic causes as well as enquiring into lifestyle and work/home circumstances. The most important component in diagnosing erectile dysfunction is to obtain a complete medical and sexual history.

Erectile dysfunction is NOT an inevitable consequence of ageing! Some may believe that a real man is looking for and desires to have sex at any time. This is not true. As a man ages, sex becomes a less important driving factor and other life factors become more important.

Scenario

A 32-year-old lawyer, Mr. Lee, comes to the Family Medicine clinic for his fatty liver follow up. At the end of the consultation, he tells you warily about his problem with his girlfriend as he has difficulties in getting an erection. He wants to know whether this is a temporary problem and whether it will affect his ability to father children in the future. On questioning it emerges that he has been with this girlfriend for 14 years (since secondary school) and has had no previous relationship. They are saving money for an endowment of an apartment and are planning to get married next year.

What are the likely diagnoses and how do you proceed to make a final diagnosis?

First of all, we need to clarify the nature of the problem from the patient

- Lack of sex drive (loss of libido)
- Failure to erect
- Failure to maintain an erection for penetration
- Premature ejaculation
- Retrograde ejaculation

The most likely causes

- Psychological disorders: depression/stressed induced

- Vascular disorders: atherosclerosis, ischaemic heart disease, peripheral vascular disease, hypertension
- Hormonal disorders: loss of libido through hypogonadism, hyper/hypothyroidism
- Metabolic disorders: diabetes mellitus, obesity, hyperlipidemia
- Neurological disorders: pelvic surgery, spinal injury, multiple sclerosis
- Habits: alcohol, smoking, marijuana/narcotics abuse
- Drug-induced: antidepressants (depress libido), antiandrogens, most antipsychotics and antihypertensives in particular thiazide diuretics

Other uncommon causes include renal failure, cerebral disease and Cushing/Addison's disease.

Sexual history checklists

About the problem
- Duration of the problem
- Time of onset
- Patient's (and partner's) ideals, concerns and expectations

About the patient
- Sexuality
- Sex education
- First intercourse
- Parental relationship
- Child abuse
- Family and personal beliefs and attitudes (including religion) towards sex, masturbation

About the relationship
- Mutual attraction
- Frequency of intercourse
- Pain or discomfort during intercourse
- Orgasm
- Worries about pregnancy, HIV/STD

Specific questions to ask that may help

- Sometimes clinicians may feel awkward and do not know how to begin asking sexual history questions. The clinician can begin by saying, "I need to ask a few short questions about your sexual health in order to be thorough in providing you with medical care." If a clinician does feel awkward it is essential that they recognise this and deal with the issue and not let it affect the consultation.

- Sexuality covers a broad spectrum and it is possible for any (apparently) heterosexual man or woman to be attracted to members of their own sex. Pressure from society, parents and the law means that people may refuse to come to terms with this and to "come out". Some can become desperately lonely and depressed, with high suicide rates. Therefore as a doctor, you should never make any assumption about anyone's sexuality. Be open and ready to talk about it. Prepare the patient and explain why it is important for you to know, and never be judgemental. You could ask some indirect questions:
  ❖ What arouses you or turns you on?
  ❖ Do you look forward to making love?
  ❖ Does making love make you happy or relaxed?

- Enquiring about possible child sexual abuse is an important part of the history. For example, "Were there any incidences which went beyond healthy shows of affection such as hugging between family members when you were young?" or "Did you have any upsetting sexual experiences during childhood and adolescence?"

- It is known that testosterone enhances sexual interest and the frequency of sexual acts; it increases the frequency of nocturnal erections but does not affect reflexogenic or psychogenic erections. It is important to ask about the nature of the problem as management will differ.

Sexual questionnaire

Several validated sexual questionnaires such as the 15-item IIEF (International Index of Erectile Function) or its 5-item abridged version, SHIM (Sexual Health Inventory for Men) (Table 22.1) and EDITS (Erectile Dysfunction Inventory of Treatment Satisfaction) allow one to detect the presence and grade the severity of erectile dysfunction.

Allowing the patient to complete such a questionnaire before his first clinical consultation may produce a more comfortable clinical environment. This will also act as a baseline for monitoring and evaluating the effectiveness of future intervention.

Examination

The physical examination should focus on the vascular, neurological and endocrine systems. Routine medical examination should include urinalysis and BP measurement. Testes size should be noted and the penis shaft examined to rule out a penile deformity (Peyronie's disease).

Investigations

Recommendations vary as to what laboratory investigations need to be done but exhaustive biochemical screening and psychological assessments no longer apply. Instead, basic screening such as haemoglobin, fasting glucose and lipid profile should be carried out. Other investigations should follow clinical suspicion of specific disorders. Hormonal screening is controversial. Screening for free testosterone will better predict the true level of testosterone available in the body but is not generally available in the local laboratory. In the case of loss of libido, abnormally low morning total testosterone level on two separate occasions may be indicative of the problem.

A number of specialised investigations such as duplex ultrasonography and selective pudendal artieriography are only required for candidates for penile revascularisation surgery, such as patients under 40 with a history of pelvic trauma and would therefore be organised by the appropriate specialist.

Table 22.1 5-item abridged version of Sexual Health Inventory for Men over the past 6 months:

1. How would you rate your **confidence** in your ability to get and keep an erection?
   - ○ Very Low
   - ○ Low
   - ○ Moderate
   - ○ High
   - ○ Very High

2. When you had erections with sexual stimulation, **how often** were your erections hard enough for penetration (entering your partner)?
   - ○ No sexual activity
   - ○ Almost never/Never
   - ○ A few times (much less than half the time)
   - ○ Sometimes (about half the time)
   - ○ Most times (much more than half the time)
   - ○ Almost always/Always

3. During sexual intercourse, **how often** were you able to maintain your erection after you had penetrated (entered) your partner?
   - ○ Did not attempt intercourse
   - ○ Almost never/Mever
   - ○ A few times (much less than half the time)
   - ○ Sometimes (about half the time)
   - ○ Most times (much more than half the time)
   - ○ Almost always/Always

4. During sexual intercourse, **how difficult** was it to maintain your erection to completion of intercourse?
   - ○ Did not attempt intercourse
   - ○ Extremely difficult
   - ○ Very difficult
   - ○ Difficult
   - ○ Slightly difficult
   - ○ Not difficult

5. When you attempted sexual intercourse, **how often** was it satisfactory for you?
   - ○ Did not attempt intercourse
   - ○ Almost never/Never
   - ○ A few times (much less than half the time)
   - ○ Sometimes (about half the time)
   - ○ Most times (much more than half the time)
   - ○ Almost always/Always

Scenario

In his follow-up visit, Mr. Lee is told that his total cholesterol is raised, body mass index (BMI) is 26.3 and total testosterone is reduced. However he confesses that he has never attempted sexual intercourse with this girlfriend by virtue of a mutual agreement to wait until they are married. He lied because he had a one-night affair with a colleague when on a business trip and failed to erect. He admits he was drinking heavily on that day. To further complicate matters, he was separated from his girlfriend briefly 2 years ago when she met someone else. At that time he started to visit sex workers when he was feeling low. He did manage intercourse with the workers but felt very guilty about it, yet he was unable to stop himself from doing it. He is still jealous and angry about the girlfriend's previous relationship. At the same time, he is worried about sexually transmitted diseases (STDs) and HIV, his helplessness in his own behaviour, and how to face his girlfriend, in addition to this accidental finding of reduced testosterone.

Management of erectile dysfunction

Telling lies about sexual behaviour

With the stigma and social condemnation associated with prostitution, few male clients would admit this habit to other people, including their doctor. This decision is taken at the risk of inappropriate diagnosis and treatment and it is unlikely to change until trust is established between the physician and patient. Family doctors have the advantage of continuity of care but, at the same time, they need to create an atmosphere to facilitate such conversation (e.g. the presence of a nurse in the consultation room may discourage disclosure of sensitive issues) and doctors must guard confidentiality rigorously.

Psychological causes that can be overcome

The most important psychogenic factors for the development and persistence of erectile impairment include one or a number of the following:

- Anticipative anxiety

- Performance orientation
- The partner's negative reaction to rare failure
- The observer's attitude
- Antisexual upbringing
- Monotony of sexual intercourse
- Persisting sexual myths and unsuitable attitudes
- Impaired communication between the couple
- Different sexual preferences
- Psychic and sexual traumas and pathological mental conditions

Moreover when a physiological cause is treated, subsequent self-esteem problems may continue to impair normal function and performance. Qualified therapists (e.g. sex counsellors, psychotherapists) work with couples to reduce tension, improve sexual communication and create realistic expectations about sex, all of which can improve erectile function.

Psychological therapy may be effective in conjunction with medical or surgical treatment. Sex therapists emphasise the need for men and their partners to be motivated and willing to adapt to psychological and behavioural modifications, including those that result from medical or surgical treatment.

Screening for HIV and STDs

HIV/STDs are thriving in this region and one survey showed that 80% of them were treated in the private sector, of which primary care was one of the three most cited. There are over 30 types of STDs. Sometimes the presence of symptoms such as colour/odour of the discharge or appearance of ulcerative lesions can indicate what to screen for. In the absence of symptoms, testing for gonorrhoea, chlamydia, syphilis and hepatitis B are recommended based on epidemiology.

Pre HIV-test counselling includes risk assessment, exploring the patient's social network, preparing the patient for a positive test, and ensuring the patient understands the basic facts of HIV/AIDS. The doctor should explain the "window period" and arrange post-test counselling. It is also a golden opportunity for educating patients in safer sexual practices.

Summary of management

In Mr. Lee's case, he seems to have a number of risk factors (alcohol, obesity, raised cholesterol) related to erectile dysfunction that need to be addressed and certainly psychosocial issues play a considerable role. He should at least have another test for testosterone and regular follow ups. He can be reassured that since he can perform "satisfactorily" with some women his problem is unlikely to be purely organic. In fact many problems of this kind have mixed aetiology and thus clinical presentation.

With the introduction of oral therapy (sildenafil, vardenafil and tadalafil), most patients with this condition are now managed in primary care. Both sildenafil and vardenafil have been shown to improve the ability to attain and maintain an erection when taken an hour before intercourse. Vardenafil distinguishes itself by demonstrating efficacy in patients who had undergone radical prostatectomy and patients with diabetes. Tadalafil exhibits a prolonged half-life (Table 22.2) and is not clinically influenced by alcohol or co-existing diseases such as diabetes or renal or hepatic impairment. Although they should not be given to patients taking nitrates because of the risk of hypotension, they are generally well-tolerated by the majority of patients including those with stable heart disease or hypertension.

Table 22.2 Pharmacokinetics of PDE-5 inhibitors

	Sildenafil 100mg	Vardenafil 20mg	Tadalafil 20mg
Tmax (hr)	1.16	0.75	2.0
T $^1/_2$ (hr)	3.8	4.7	17.5

Summary

Despite the fact that erectile dysfunction can have a dramatically negative impact on a man's sense of well-being, it is often undiagnosed and under-treated. Breaking the ice by both doctors and patients is an essential first step. Better training and ready use of oral PDE-5 agents would transform the treatment of erectile dysfunction in primary care.

Notes

1. P. Mariappan and W. L. Chong. "Prevalence and correlations of lower urinary tract symptos, erectile dysfunction and incontinence in men from a multiethnic Asian population: Results of a regional population-based survey and comparison with industrialized nations". *BJU International*, 98 (6): 1264–1268, December 2006.
2. J. Prins, M. H. Blanker, A. M. Bohnen, S. Thomas and J. L. Bosch. "Prevalence of erectile dysfunction: A systematic review of population-based studies". *International Journal of Impotence Research*, 14 (6): 422–432, December 2002.
3. M. K. Li, L. A. Garcia and R. Rosen. "Lower urinary tract symptoms and male sexual dysfunction in Asia: A survey of ageing men from five Asian countries". *BJU International*, 96 (9): 1339–1354, December 2005.

Chapter 23

Menstrual Problems

♦ William C. W. WONG ♦

In Hong Kong, women presenting with reproductive problems constitute a significant part of a family doctor's workload (around 2% in young adults of 20–44 years old) (Lee et al. 1994). There is wide variability among women in terms of cycle length, perceived and actual menstrual blood loss, and regularity of bleeding. What one woman perceives as "normal" can be regarded as "unacceptable" by another. Hence, given the subjectivity of many of the symptoms associated with menstruation, the doctor's first task is to determine whether or not their symptoms indicate any underlying pathology which warrants further management. Only when this is established can the patient's concerns be addressed and advice offered, and often in this way unnecessary investigation can be avoided.

Scenario

Lei Ming, a 34-year-old clerk working for a busy trading company, saw her family doctor for the first time and complained of secondary amenorrhoea. Her first menarche started at age 13 and she has had irregular menstrual periods ever since. Her menstrual cycle usually varies between 26 and 60 days. However her last menstrual period was 4 months ago. She had done a few pregnancy tests which were consistently negative.

What are the likely diagnoses and how do you proceed to make a final diagnosis?

The most likely causes

- Polycystic ovary syndrome (PCOS)
- Menopause including premature ovarian failure
- Severe emotional distress

The important possibilities that (may) need to be excluded

- Endocrine disorders: thyroid disease, adrenal disease
- Physiological: rapid weight loss, excessive exercise/training
- Anorexia nervosa

The rare or unusual possibilities

- Prolactinoma and other pituitary tumours
- Pituitary failure

Features of the history that may help differentiate between possible causes of her irregular periods

Many women during their reproductive years may fixate on having regular, predictable periods. Changes in the pattern of menstruation often invoke anxiety. The root of this anxiety may be fear of pregnancy or fear of loss of fertility with concomitant loss of femininity. Careful exploration of a woman's ideas and concerns is very important when assessing menstrual problems.

- Excessive facial hair, acne and obesity is suggestive of PCOS
- Hot flushes and night sweats are common symptoms of the menopause. Failing oestrogen production results in reflex over-production of follicular stimulating hormone (FSH) resulting in vasodilatation. It is often accompanied by palpitation and sweating, usually lasting for a few minutes
- Recent loss of weight. This can be intended, a consequence of severe emotional distress, an indication of anorexia nervosa, or be caused by hyperthyroidism. A BMI of 19 or less is thought to be necessary for amenorrhoea

- Emotional distress. Stress, for example a marital or family crisis or problems at work, can lead to amenorrhoea
- Galactorrhoea suggests prolactinoma

Examination

Examination is rarely helpful in determining the cause of irregular periods.

Investigations

- Serum gonadotrophin (FSH and LH) levels should be measured. These are normal if the cause is physiological or stress. High FSH and LH levels are found in menopause. Polycystic ovary syndrome may give an elevated LH
- Serum prolactin is raised with a prolactinoma and occasionally with PCOS
- PCOS often causes raised serum testosterone and androstenedione
- Thyroid function tests should be performed routinely to exclude thyroid disease in women of this age group and clinical presentation
- Pelvic ultrasound can reveal multiple small ovarian follicles in PCOS

Management of menstrual problems

Managing a patient with premature menopause calls for an understanding of both the biology of menopause and the impact of this diagnosis on the patient and their life. A patient-centred approach, which focuses upon identifying and addressing those issues of most significance and concern for each patient, is likely to be most helpful.

Referral is rarely necessary to establish the reason for irregular periods. However the management of some of the causes of secondary amenorrhoea may involve our colleagues in secondary care.

Scenario

Lei Ming had not been stressed or distressed lately, indeed she has recently embarked on a new relationship in which she is very happy. Her weight has been stable (BMI = 22). Serum gonadotrophin levels revealed elevated FSH and LH suggesting she is peri-menopausal. She was then referred to a gynaecologist for further assessment.

Lei Ming is young and has recently embarked on a new relationship. For her, the psychological and emotional implications of the diagnosis may be quite profound. Premature menopause brings with it probable infertility. This may be devastating for Lei Ming personally as she probably hopes to become a mother in the future, and be potentially destructive for present and future relationships. In contrast, for women who have completed their family, issues of infertility may be of secondary importance to the physical consequences of premature ovarian failure, such as osteoporosis, and to the psychological effects of feeling "old before their time".

Effective management of patients with premature menopause requires doctors to exercise a wide range of skills.

Empathy

Patients want doctors to be able to appreciate their perspective on their illness and to show compassion and understanding for this perspective. Being empathetic can provide patients with much comfort in situations such as this in which cure is not possible.

Explanation

Helping patients to understand their diagnosis and its consequences is an important aspect of management of the menopause. For most women with premature menopause, the cause is never identified. Of the known causes auto-immune disorders, genetic factors and endocrine disorders (thyroid disorders, diabetes and pituitary problems) are most common along with iatrogenic causes. The physical, psychological and social implications of the menopause should be discussed.

Referral

The ovarian failure of premature menopause may be incomplete and a minority of women may ovulate occasionally. Referral to specialist gynaecology services for tracking of ovarian activity may be indicated.

Support/Self-help groups

Support can be gained from sharing experiences with other women in similar circumstances. This support can be obtained through attending groups or through, for example, Internet chat rooms.

Prescribing

Patients with premature menopause are at increased risk of developing osteoporosis. Hormone replacement therapy is an effective prophylactic treatment after balancing its risks and side-effects. Prescription should occur after a full discussion of the risks and benefits with the patient so she can make an informed choice about treatment. Local application of vaginal estrogen cream once daily for a week can provide dramatic symptomatic improvement for atrophy of the urogenital organs.

For menorrhagia, intravenous conjugated estrogen or intra-myometrial tranxenamic acid followed by oral tranxenamic acid +/– progestrogen will usually stop the bleeding. If they fail to do so one may consider dilatation and curettage of the uterus as a diagnostic and therapeutic treatment. Use of endometrial thermal balloon and microwave are still experimental. Endometrial ablation is out of fashion because of the high recurrence rate. Progestrogen IUCD cannot relieve acute menorrhagia.

For prolonged spotting (which is common in the perimenopausal period) due to progestrogen insufficiency and anovulation, 10 to 12 days of progestrogen taken in the second half of the cycle can regulate the pattern. Hysteroscopy +/– dilatation and curettage of the uterus for persistent cases may pick up some subtle intra-uterine pathology.

Counselling

Doctors are often able to support women through early menopause. For some patients, the diagnosis may raise issues for which specialist counselling might be helpful. It is important to recognise when women could potentially benefit from such approaches and facilitate appropriately their access to such services.

Opportunistic screening and education

Screen for cervical cancer using PAP smear, conduct breast examination and advise on mammogram.

Epilogue

Lei Ming was referred to the gynaecologist for ovarian tracking, but no ovarian activity was detected. She visited her family doctor on a number of occasions to discuss her feelings about her infertility. They also discussed hormone replacement therapy. Six months after being diagnosed, Lei Ming started on HRT with good support from her boyfriend.

Reference

Lee, A., Chan, K. K. C., Wun, Y. T., Ma, P. L., Li, L. and Siu, P. C. 1995. "A morbidity survey in Hong Kong, 1994". *The Hong Kong Practitioner*, 17: 246–255.

Chapter 24

Fever in Young Children

✎

◆ Albert LEE ◆

Fever is one of most common reasons why parents bring their children to family doctors. In Hong Kong, fever accounts for around 10% of attendance at Accident and Emergency Departments among those aged 9 years or under (Lee et al. 2001). Fever in infants is defined as a rectal temperature above 38°C (100°F), and in older children as a rectal temperature of 38.4°C (101°F) or oral temperature of 37.8°C (Green 1998). Although fever is mostly associated with self-limiting viral illness, it will be a presenting feature of serious bacterial infections such as meningitis, urinary tract infection and pneumonia. The younger the child, the less obvious the signs and symptoms are. Family doctors in primary health care cannot perform a full septic screen for all children with fever because of the high volume of fever cases, discomfort to the children, financial costs and potential consequences of false positive results as against the small risk of a serious bacterial infection. Therefore family doctors are often put in a difficult position when confronted with these common but ambiguous cases, in addition coping as in this case with a worried and unsupported parent.

Scenario

An anxious mother is waiting outside your clinic when you re-open for the afternoon. She claims that her 3-month-old son (her first and only child) has had a high temperature for a day. She moved to a public estate in Tin Shui Wai with her husband recently and all her friends and relatives live quite far from her. It is the first time you meet her and the child.

What are the likely diagnoses and how do you proceed to make a final diagnosis?

The most likely causes

- Viral respiratory infection
- Acute otitis media
- Gastroenteritis

The important possibilities that (may) need to be excluded

- Meningitis
- Pneumonia
- Urinary tract infection

Low risk criteria

Accurate assessment of degree of wellness for infants under 3 months old is difficult and they are at greater risk of serious infection. In the past there was a tendency to admit them to hospital for sepsis evaluation and to receive broad spectrum antibiotics pending the results of culture (Jones and Bass 1993). However this approach can be very expensive and exposes the child and the family to potential untoward sequelae of hospital admission (Levy 1979). Many studies now show that only a small proportion of febrile infants younger than 3 months who fit low-risk criteria will suffer from occult bacterial infection (Baraff 2000; Baker et al. 1999; Chiu et al. 1997; Jaskiewicz et al. 1994; Baker et al. 1993; Broner et al. 1990; Dagan et al. 1985, 1988). See Table 24.1.

Table 24.1 Low risk criteria of fever in infants

Clinical Criteria	Laboratory Criteria
• Full term ($\geq$ 37 weeks) with no complications • Previously healthy • No toxic manifestation* • No focal bacterial infection (except otitis media)	• White blood cell count 5–15×10^9/l, < 1.5×10^9 band cells/l, or band/neutrophil ratio < 2 • Normal urinalysis results such as negative gram stain of unspun urine, negative leucocyte esterase and nitrite, fewer than five white blood cells per high power field

Clinical Criteria	Laboratory Criteria
* Toxic is defined as a clinical picture consistent with the sepsis syndrome (i.e. lethargy, signs of poor perfusion, or marked hypoventilation or cyanosis). Lethargy means altered level of consciousness characterised by poor or absent eye contact or failure of interaction with persons or objects in the environment, particularly inability to recognise parents	• If diarrhoea is present, no haem and < 5wbc per high power field < 8×10^6 wbc/l in CSF and negative gram stain if lumbar puncture is performed • No infiltrate on chest X-ray

Specific questions to ask that may help

- Ask about the infant's condition before fever such as level of activities (playing with toys or interested in things), eating and drinking patterns, and any unusual behaviour as fever alone sometimes makes a child appear toxic

- Any vomiting or diarrhoea

- Number of wet diapers (to assess level of hydration)

- Past medical history including birth history and post-natal history

- Immunisation history

- Contact with ill individuals/current health status of family members

- History of recent travel or visits

- Most mothers will give a very clear indication of the seriousness of the child's illness. Phrases such as "I've never seen him like this" should be taken seriously and her concerns explored.

Examination

General

A complete physical examination with special emphasis on hydration status and an attempt to identify a possible source of infection. The physical examination should also include the vital signs such as pulse, respiratory rate and if applicable blood pressure. Accurate body weight must be recorded or charted on a growth chart.

The family doctor should look for:

- A toxic appearance such as signs of lethargy, poor perfusion, hypoventilation or hyperventilation, cyanosis, pale-looking or any symptoms or signs suggesting shock

- Any focus of infection including otitis media, pharyngitis, sinusitis and skin of soft tissue infection

- Any identifiable infection such as bronchiolitis, cramp, gingivostomatitis, viral gastroenteritis, varicella-zoster virus or hand-foot-and-mouth diseases

- Any rash particularly petechia or purpura which are often associated with invasive bacteraemia.

After the history and examination, a working diagnosis of fever without source of infection is reached. About 20% of infants will have fever without source of infection after evaluation of history and clinical assessment (Lee and Harper 1998; Soman 1985). The question now is how the doctor should communicate with the mother and how the child should be managed.

Investigations

As we can see, to assess the level of risk some simple blood tests are required which can be difficult to obtain for a young child in the family practice setting. Nevertheless, after thorough assessment, if the infant (aged 1–3 months) is of low risk without any focus of infection, he might not need to be admitted to hospital, provided that he receives good care from his carers and has easy access to the family doctor. The key question to ask at this stage is whether lumbar puncture is required for infants below

3 months with fever. Five publications reported the results of low-risk laboratory criteria without lumbar puncture in 872 low-risk infants: Only ten (1.1%) had serious bacterial infection and none had meningitis (Chiu et al. 1997; Jaskiewicz et al. 1994; Dagan et al. 1988; Anbar et al. 1986). Therefore it can be withheld unless empirical antibiotics are given. A less conservative approach may be required (e.g. referral to the local paediatric unit). This will depend upon the care provided by the local practice and the family.

Management of fever in young children

Neonates have a greater risk of systematic infections and haematogenous spread of infection. Moreover the symptoms and signs are more subtle in neonates. Even those with a clear source of infection still carry a significant risk of sepsis and meningitis with serious consequences in terms of morbidity and mortality. Thorough evaluation with complete sepsis evaluation should include a culture of cerebrospinal fluid, blood and urine; a complete blood count and differential count; examination of cerebrospinal fluid for cells, glucose and protein; and urinalysis (Baraff et al. 1993). Although in the past it was suggested that all infants under one month old be hospitalised with complete sepsis evaluation and parental antimicrobial therapy, careful observation without therapy pending culture results could be another option, especially in selected "low risk" cases as described above.

Management decision for those aged 3–36 months old is mainly based on the degree of toxicity and the level of fever. They can be managed in an outpatient setting if they fulfill the following criteria:

- Child was well prior to onset of fever
- Child's fever is $< 39°C$
- Child has no significant risk factors
- Child appears non-toxic and otherwise healthy
- Child's laboratory results are within reference ranges defined as low risk (Table 24.1)
- Parents appear reliable and have access to family doctors easily

Nevertheless the main difficulty is to decide what laboratory tests should be performed in the primary care setting to identify an "occult infection" such as urinary tract infection, pneumonia, bacteraemia or meningitis. As viral infections are far more prevalent than bacterial infections, the positive predictive value of elevated WBC count for occult bacterial infection is rather low (8–15% in most studies) (Kramer and Shapiro 1997). Most young febrile children with high WBC count do not have an underlying bacterial infection as the cause of fever (Kramer and Shapiro 1997). Even among the true positives, most will have an infection that will resolve spontaneously or respond to treatment without serious sequelae even if not diagnosed earlier. The positive predictive value for most serious infections is many times lower. Therefore family doctors may not need to rush to perform invasive blood tests at the initial stage for this category of children.

How to rule out occult UTI

UTI is among the most common occult bacterial infection in children (especially in girls), i.e. in nearly 5% of febrile infants under 12 months old and in 2% of febrile children under 5 years old (AAP 1999; Shaw et al. 1998; Hoberman et al. 1993). The risk is higher among those with high fever and without source of infection (Hoberman and Wald 1997). The prevalence is greater in boys younger than 6 months than in those between 6 to 12 months (2.7% vs. 1.3%). In a study of 4,255 children less than 24 months old, the use of "enhanced urinalysis" for the presence of pyuria (defined as 10 or more WBC) had sensitivity of 95.8%, a specificity of 92.6%, and thus a positive predictive value of 40.4% (Hobernam et al. 1996, 1997, 1999). Shaw et al. reported that urine with negative "urine dipstick" was unlikely to generate a positive urine culture. In the case of younger girls or uncircumcised boys < 6–12 months a urine culture will probably be required. This will replace routine urine culture for all young children with high fever as a sample obtained by catherisation or suprapubic aspiration can result in discomfort and the procedure is invasive for young children. A negative urinalysis on a clean catch specimen is sufficient to replace urine culture in assessment of children with fever in most cases.

How to rule out occult pneumonia

The majority of pneumonias in infants and young children are non-bacterial and caused by virus (Boyer and Cherry 1992; Turner et al. 1987). Bacterial infections sometimes occur as a secondary infection after an initial respiratory viral infection. Studies have shown that only 3% of infants and young children without tachypnoea, respiratory distress, rales or decreased breathing sounds had occult pneumonia (Baraff et al. 1993; Singal et al. 1989; Zukin et al. 1986). A study reported that 26% of children with fever (39°C or higher) and a WBC 20,000/mm^3 or higher without source of infection had radiographic evidence of pneumonia (Bachur et al. 1999). Therefore chest X-ray can be considered for children with a fever of 39.5°C, a WBC of 20,000/mm^3 or higher, a normal urinalysis and who have not had a streptococcous pneumonae vaccination.

How to rule out occult bacteraemia

The risk of occult bacteraemia in all non-toxic infants and young children without source of infection with temperature of 39°C or higher is between 2.6% to 6.1% (Fleisher et al. 1994; Bass et al. 1993; Jaffee et al. 1987). Risk increases with higher temperature. In the majority of children occult pnemococcal bacteraemia resolves without therapy (Baraff 2000), but studies show the risk of bacterial meningitis to be 4% in the no antibiotics group, i.e. those with no source of infection treated as outpatients without antibiotics. In view of the low risk of occult bacteraemia in children with temperature less than 39.5°C, and even lower risk in children with temperature greater than 39.5°C and WBC less than 15,000/mm^3, Baraff (2000) has revised the practice guideline by raising the threshold for obtaining a screening WBC count to 39.5°C.

Decision-making in management

Based on an understanding of the epidemiology of occult infections, the management decision will take into account the temperature and degree of toxicity. The Yale Observation Scale is a reliable method for determining the degree of severity of illness (Bonadio 1998; Teach and Fleish 1995; McCarthy et al. 1985). It consists of 6 variables: quality of cry, reaction to parent stimulation, state variation, colour, hydration and response (Table 24.2). A score of 10 or less has 2.7% risk of serious bacterial infection and a score of 16 or greater has a 92% risk of serious bacterial infection. The scale provides additional information in decision-making in clinical management of children aged 3 to 36 months with fever. Figure 24.1 summarises as an algorithm the management of a healthy child aged 3 to 36 months by family doctors in the primary care setting.

A toxic-looking child will need the appropriate culture and diagnostic tests, hospitalisation and antibiotics treatment (preferably via the parental route). If no focus of infection is found in a child who appears well and

Table 24.2 Summary of the Yale Observation Scale

Observation Items	1 (Normal)	3 (Moderate Impairment)	5 (Severe Impairment)
Quality of cry	Strong with normal tone or contentment without crying	Whimpering or sobbing	Weak cry, moaning or high-pitched cry
Reaction to parent stimulation	Brief crying that stops or contentment without crying	Intermittent crying	Continual crying or limited response
Colour	Pink	Acrocyanotic or pale extremities	Pale or cyanotic or mottled or ashen
State variation	If awake, stays awake; if asleep, wakes up quickly upon stimulation	Eyes closed briefly while awake or awake with prolonged stimulation	Falls asleep or will not arouse
Hydration	Skin normal, eyes normal and mucous membranes moist	Skin and eyes normal and mouth slightly dry	Skin doughy or tented, dry mucous membranes and/or sunken eyes
Response (e.g. talk, smile) to social overtures	Smiling or alert (< 2 months)	Briefly smiling or alert briefly (< 2 months)	Unsmiling anxious face or dull, expressionless, or not alert (< 2 months)

fulfills the low risk criteria, no diagnostic tests other than urinalysis will be needed. No antibiotics should be given. Close monitoring will allow a subsequent change of clinical management should the condition deteriorate. If the competency of carers is in doubt, the family doctor may consider admission or repeated observation over time.

If the child develops any of the following conditions, it becomes an emergency case and the child will benefit from hospital admission:

- Parents have observed deterioration of condition as described above but are unable to contact the family doctor
- Dehydration

Figure 24.1 Algorithm for fever management in children aged 3 to 36 months with no source of infection

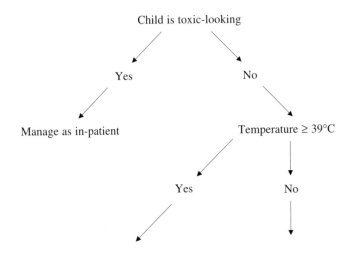

Child is toxic-looking

Yes   No

Manage as in-patient   Temperature ≥ 39°C

Yes   No

1. For males ≤ 6 months and uncircumcised, males 6–12 months, female < 12 months, urine culture.

2. For circumcised males 6–12 months and all females 12–24 months, microscopic urinalysis or urine dipstick (leukocyte esterase and nitrite), if possible urine culture.

3. For fever ≥ 39.5°C, obtain WBC count; if ≥ 15,000 or absolute neutrophil count ≥ 10,000, send blood culture.

4. Chest X-ray if respiratory distress, tachypnoea rates or temperature ≥ 39°C and WBC count > 20,000.

5. Paracetamol 15mg/kg q4h for fever.

6. Consult again if fever persists > 48 hours or if condition deteriorates.

a. No diagnostic work up or antibiotics.

b. Paracetamol 15mg/kg/dose q6h for fever.

c. Return if fever persists > 48 hours or if condition deteriorates.

Source: Baraff 2000

- Seizure
- Development of rash
- Change of consciousness level
- Dyspnoea with shallow, rapid or difficult breathing
- Severe vomiting
- Persistent diarrhoea
- Persistent headache

The optimum care for childhood fever really depends on the condition under which the child seeks help. Lack of previous contacts with the child and family in an emergency department or tertiary institution, and uncertainty about the adequacy of parental surveillance and compliance with follow ups, will make a doctor feel that there is only one opportunity to make the correct diagnosis and initiate treatment (Schriger 1997; Kramer and Shapiro 1997). Family doctors with a long established relationship with the family and easy accessibility have more than one opportunity to act if the child's condition changes. Studies cited in previous sections have shown that there is sufficient time to treat the majority of children with fever before their condition deteriorates if they are not toxic-ooking at initial presentation. Diagnostic testing and "blind" treatment are poor substitutes for good family medical care. Family doctors should teach the carers to recognise the "sinister" symptoms and signs. It is unlikely that more aggressive management will substantially decrease population-based rates of meningitis or sepsis in young children, because these conditions are rare in a population.

Summary

Fever is one of the commonest health problems for general practice consultation for children. It is also one of the main reasons why parents take their children to Accident and Emergency departments. Most young children with fever and no focus of infection present with self-limiting viral illness and disappear without sequela. Only a few children may develop occult bacteraemia that may be associated with serious bacterial infection. The dilemma for family doctors in differentiating those children with serious infection from self-limiting conditions in primary care setting. Careful clinical assessment including all relevant history and clinical examination supplemented by basic laboratory tests if needed, and careful monitoring of changes in symptoms and signs are the keys in management to avoid the risks of misdiagnosis of serious conditions or over investigations and treatments. Family doctors also need to education parents and carers to be more vigilant in the observation of possible early warning symptoms and signs of serious clinical conditions so that prompt medical attention would be given.

References

American Academy of Pediatrics, Committee on Quality Improvement, Subcommittee on Urinary Tract Infection. 1999. "Practice parameter: The diagnosis, treatment, and evaluation of the initial urinary tract infection in febrile infants and young children". *Pediatrics*, 103: 843–852.

Anbar, R. D., Richardson-del, C. V. and O'Malley, P. J. 1986. "Difficulties in universal application of criteria identifying infants at low risk for serious bacterial infection". *Journal of Pediatrics*, 109: 483–485.

Bachur, R., Perry, H. and Harper, M. B. 1999. "Occult pneumonias: Empiric chest radiographs in febrile children with leukocytosis". *Annals of Emergency Medicine*, 33: 166–173.

Baker, M. D., Bell, L. M. and Avner, J. R. 1993. "Outpatient management without antibiotics of fever in selected infants". *New England Journal of Medicine*, 329: 1437–1441.

———. 1999. "The efficacy of routine outpatient management without antibiotics of fever in selected infants". *Pediatrics*, 103: 627–631.

Baraff, L. J. 2000. "Management of fever without source in infants and children". *Annals of Emergency Medicine*, 36: 602–614.

Baraff, L. J., Bass, J. W., Fleisher, G. R., Klein, J. O., McCracken, G. H., Powell, K. R. and Schriger, D. L. 1993. "Practice guideline for the management of infants and children 0 to 36 months of age with fever without source". *Pediatrics*, 92: 1–12.

Bass, J. W., Steele, R. W., Wittler, R. R., et al. 1993. "Antimicrobial treatment of occult bacteremia: A multicenter cooperative study". *Pediatric Infectious Disease Journal*, 12: 466–473.

Bonadio, W. A. 1998. "The history and physical assessments of the febrile infant". *Pediatric Clinics of North America*, 45 (1): 65–77.

Boyer, K. M. and Cherry, J. D. 1992. "Nonbacterial pneumonia". In R. D. Feigin and J. D. Cherry (eds.), *Textbook of Pediatric Infectious Disease*. Philadelphia: WB Saunders, pp. 254–265.

Broner, C. W., Polk, S. A. and Sherman, J. M. 1990. "Febrile infants less than eight weeks old: Predictors of infection". *Clinical Pediatrics*, 29: 438–443.

Chiu, C. H., Lin, T. Y. and Bullard, M. J. 1997. "Identification of febrile neonates unlikely to have bacterial infections". *Pediatric Infectious Disease Journal*, 16: 59–63.

Dagan, R., Powell, K. R., Hall, C. B., et al. 1985. "Identification of infants unlikely to have serious bacterial infection although hospitalised for suspected sepsis". *Journal of Pediatrics*, 107: 855–860.

Dagan, R., Sofer, S., Phillip, M., et al. 1988. "Ambulatory care of febrile infants younger than 2 months of age classified as being at low risk for having serious bacterial infections". *Journal of Pediatrics*, 112: 355–360.

Fleisher, G. R., Rosenberg, N., Vinci, R., et al. 1994. "Intramuscular versus oral antibiotic therapy for the prevention of meningitis and other bacterial sequelae in young, febrile children at risk for occult bacteremia". *Journal of Pediatrics*, 124: 504–512.

Green, M. 1998. "Fever". In *Pediatric Diagnosis*. Philadelphia: WB Saunders, p. 203.

Hoberman, A., Chao, H. P., Keller, D. M., et al. 1993. "Prevalence of urinary tract infection in febrile infants". *Journal of Pediatrics*, 123: 17–23.

Hoberman, A., Wald, E. R., Penchansky, L., et al. 1993. "Enhanced urinalysis as a screening test for urinary tract infection". *Pediatrics*, 91: 1196–1199.

Hoberman, A., Wald, E. R., Reynolds, E. A., et al. 1996. "Is urine culture necessary to rule out urinary tract infection in young febrile children?". *Pediatric Infectious Disease Journal*, 15: 304–309.

Hoberman, A. and Wald, E. R. 1997. "Urinary tract infections in young febrile infants". *Pediatric Infectious Disease Journal*, 16: 11–17.

Hoberman, A., Wald, E. R., Hickey, R. W., Baskin, M., Charron, M., Majd, M., Kearney, D. H., Reynolds, E. A., Ruley, J. and Janosky, J. E. 1999. "Oral versus initial intravenous therapy for urinary tract infections in young febrile children". *Pediatrics*, 104: 79–86.

Jaffe, D. M., Tanz, R. R., Davis, A. T., et al. 1987. "Antibiotics administration to treat possible occult bacteraemia in febrile children". *New England Journal of Medicine,* 317: 1157–1180.

Jaskiewicz, J. A., McCarthy, C. A., Richardson, A. C., et al. 1994. "Febrile infants at low risk for serious bacterial infection—An appraisal of the Rochester criteria and implications for management". *Pediatrics*, 94: 390–396.

Jones, R. G. and Bass, J. W. 1993. "Febrile children with no focus of infection: A survey of their management by primary care physicians". *Pediatric Infectious Disease Journal*, 12: 179–183.

Kramer, M. S. and Shapiro, E. D. 1997. "Management of the young febrile child: A commentary on recent practice guidelines". *Pediatrics*, 100: 128–134.

Lee, A., Lau, F. L., Hazlett, C. B., Kam, C. W., Wong, P., Wong, T. W. and Chow, S., 2001. "Analysis of the morbidity pattern of non-urgent patients attending accident and emergency departments in Hong Kong". *Hong Kong Medical Journal*, 7: 311–318.

Lee, G. M. and Harper, M. B. 1998. "Risk of bacteremia for febrile young children in the post-Haemophilus influenzae type b era". *Archives of Pediatrics and Adolescent Medicine*, 152: 624–628.

Levy, J. C. 1979. "Vulnerable children: Parents' perspectives and use of medical care". *Pediatrics*, 65: 956–963.

McCarthy, P. L., Lembo, R. M., Buron, M. A., Fink, H. D. and Cicchetti, D. V. 1985. "Predicitve value of abnormal physical examination findings in ill appearing and well appearing febrile children". *Pediatrics*, 76 (2): 167–171.

Schriger, D. L. 1997. "Management of the young febrile child. Clinical guidelines in the setting of incomplete evidence [commentary]". *Pediatrics*, 100: 136.

Shaw, K. N., Gorelick, M., McGowan, K. L., Yakscoe, N. McDaniel and Schwartz, J. S. 1998, "Prevalence of urinary tract infection in febrile young children in the emergency department". *Pediatrics*, 102.e16. Available at: http://www.pediatrics.org/cgi/contents/full/102/2/e16.

Singal, B. M., Hedges, J. R. and Radack, K. L. 1989. "Decision rules and clinical prediction of pneumonia: Evaluation of low-yield criteria". *Annals of Emergency Medicine*, 18: 13–20.

Soman, M. 1985. "Characteristics and management of febrile young children seen in a university family practice". *Journal of Family Practice*, 21: 117–122.

Teach, S. J. and Fleisher, G. R. 1995, "Efficacy of an observation scale in detecting bacteremia in febrile children three to thirty-six months of age, treated as outpatients". Occult Bacteremia Study Group.

Turner, R. B., Lande, A. E., Chase, P., et al. 1987. "Pneumonia in pediatric outpatients: Cause and clinical manifestations". *Journal of Pediatrics*, 111: 194–200.

Zukin, D. D., Hoffman, J. R., Cleveland, R. H., et al. 1986. "Correlation of pulmonary signs and symptoms with chest radiographs in the pediatric age group". *Annals of Emergency Medicine*, 15: 792–796.

SECTION IV

✑

Self-assessment

Self-assessment

Mr. Tim Lee is married to Nancy aged 20. A year later, they have a son, Stephen. Mrs. Lee now complains of a loss of ten pounds in body-weight in two months. Her past health has been good. She has given up her work as a secretary after giving birth to Stephen. During the previous week, she has brought Stephen to you twice for upper respiratory traction infection.

What are the possible causes of her weight loss?

Physical

– exertion

– chronic infection, e.g. TB

– thyrotoxicosis

– diabetes mellitus

– collagen vascular disease

– malabsorption

– uraemia

– chronic liver disease

– malignancy

Psychological

– anxiety

– depression

– anorexia nervosa

– alcohol/drug abuse

How can you establish the diagnosis?

History

– is the patient dieting?

– any change in everyday workload, rest, sleep, appetite

- symptoms of diabetes, thyrotoxicosis, fever, night sweat, haemoptysis, contact with TB, diarrhoea, constipation, urine habits
- mood change, thought content
- any social problems (family relations, housing, child care)
- what does she think is the cause?

Examination

- signs of weight loss, objective weight measurement, any difference as compared to previously recorded weight, body mass index
- full examination with special attention to fever, pallor, lymphadenopathy, rash, tremor, thyrotoxic eye signs, thyroid enlargement and bruit, abdominal examination, pelvic examination and mood

Investigation guided by history and examination

- may defer investigation until further observation
- initial investigations may include urine dipstick for albumin, sugar, specific gravity; CBC, ESR, LFT, RFT, fasting/spot sugar, thyroid function, X-Ray chest, stool for occult blood
- further investigations may include other endocrine function tests, barium studies or IVP

Assessment 2

Initial investigations reveal no abnormality. One week later she comes for follow up. She tells you that she has been unable to sleep for three consecutive nights. Her eyes are congested and she speaks slowly with a low-tone voice.

What do you want to discuss with her?

Investigation results

- reassure that there is no evidence of organic disease
- discuss possible causes of weight loss; review diet, rest, daily activity, mood, worries
- offer support and follow up on body weight

Insomnia

(a) history

− be empathetic, let her ventilate

− history of medication especially hypnotic

− previous sleep pattern or insomnia

− nature of insomnia: difficulty in falling asleep, frequent wakening or early morning wakening

− sleep environment: warmth, ventilation, baby crying, husband snoring

− physical symptoms: pain, cough, nocturia; associated symptoms like appetite, mood, drive, sense of worthlessness, crying episodes, suicidal tendency

− family history of sleep disorder, family relationship

(b) advice

− reassure that her health will not be damaged by a few days' lack of sleep

− get out of bed if not sleepy as lying in bed worrying about difficulty in falling asleep will only create a vicious cycle

− simple measures like soft music, hot drinks, and avoid alcohol, coffee or tea in the evening

− discourage daytime nap

− encourage exercise

− offer family therapy or counselling

Mood change

explore

− her ideas of possible causes of insomnia, her worries, expectation from consultation

− coping ability with son, household

Plan of management

− discourage hypnotic: disadvantages and side-effects explained

− psychotherapy for a pre-determined period and consider referral to social worker or psychiatrist

– consider antidepressant or tranquilliser

– follow ups for progress and further counselling

Assessment 3

Tim comes the next day, very concerned about his wife's investigations and asks you about the results. He also complains of epigastric pain which has increased in severity for the past one month, and he has been having three to four loose motions every day.

How would you conduct this consultation?

Explore true reason of consultation: Does he come for epigastric pain or to find out about his wife's problem?

Mrs. Lee's investigation

(Good opportunity to assess family dynamics and communication)

– a problem of confidentiality

– explore Tim' reason of concern

(invite Tim to provide information about his wife rather than revealing information to him)

– explore his knowledge and idea about Mrs. Lee's condition

– encourage him to talk with Mrs. Lee to find out more

Mr. Lee's epigastric pain and loose stool

(a) history

– pain: onset, duration, character, relation to meals, radiation, hunger pain, nocturnal pain, periodicity, aggravating and relieving factors, family history

– loose stool: past bowel habit, blood, mucus, travel history, appetite, weight loss, alcohol, smoking

– any stress at work or pain interfering with work

– relationship with wife, or any family problem

– finance situation

- his interpretation of the symptoms
- fear of organic disease, cancer, any anxiety or worries

(b) examination

- general signs of weight loss, fever, jaundice, palm, lymph node, abdominal examination including rectal examination or proctoscopy

(c) investigation

- depends on the pathology suspected

(d) management

- explain to him the provisional diagnosis, psychological component and management plan
- reassurance and support
- prescription according to working diagnosis

Assessment 4

The couple has not turned up since then. Two months later, Mrs. Lee brings Stephen, aged two, to you because of intermittent cough for a month. The cough becomes worse in spite of over-the-counter cough mixtures. He has not been eating well and cries every night as the cough is usually more frequent during night time thus waking him up.

What are the likely diagnoses and how are you going to manage Stephen's cough?

Possible causes

- asthma
- catarrhal child, post-nasal drip, allergic rhinitis
- foreign body inhalation
- whooping cough
- pulmonary TB
- psittacosis

–   congenital heart disease (should be known before)

–   emotional problem

–   attention seeking

Find the cause

(a) history

–   past history of cough/bronchitis

–   mode of onset, fever

–   wheeze, shortness of breath

–   eating peanuts or playing with small objects

–   smoker in family, birds or other pets, plants,

–   atopic features in Stephen and other relatives

–   relation to exercise or change of weather

–   aggravating factors

(b) examination

–   temperature, clubbing, cyanosis, accessory respiratory muscle

–   chest deformity, air entry, wheeze, crepitation

–   heart

–   growth percentile

(not possible to measure peak flow rate at age 2)

(c) investigation

–   X-ray chest to exclude foreign body or TB

–   nasal swab for whooping cough

Assess effect of cough

–   Stephen's feeding, sleep activity and growth

–   Mrs. Lee's coping, worry, frustration, guilt feelings

–   Mr. Lee's reaction

Assessment 5

Nancy (Mrs. Lee) mentions that she is going to become crazy and that she does not want to live any longer. She then bursts into tears and complains that her husband has been staying out late recently. He sleeps in his study as he is very annoyed by Stephen's crying at night.

How would you respond?

Calm Nancy down, be empathetic and give her time to ventilate.

Explore
- what she means by becoming crazy
- exact reason why she is so upset. Is it due to stress in the care of Stephen, the lack of understanding or support from husband?
- enquire about sexual problem and marital problem
- assess her feeling towards Stephen and her husband
- whether there is any hallucination, thought disorder, suicidal thought or attempts
- elicit any other symptoms of depression
- is she taking drugs or alcohol?

Counsel her on
- the cause of her distress, the possible solutions
- her attitude
- how to promote support from relatives or close friends

Support Nancy; may offer to see Mr. Lee if he agrees to come.

Prescribe antidepressant.

Referral to hospital if suicide is imminent, Samaritans, family counsellors, paediatrician.

Assess risk to Stephen on child abuse/neglect.

Admit Stephen to ease the family tension.

Arrange follow up for further development.

Assessment 6

You diagnose asthma in Stephen and the symptoms are controlled by your treatment. However, during one subsequent consultation you find that Mr. Lee has moved out for five months. According to Mrs. Lee a divorce seems inevitable.

What problems do you anticipate?

Mrs. Lee

- stress from pending divorce
- need to face relatives and friends
- increased risk of depression and suicide as a reaction to loss, anxiety and uncertainty about life ahead
- caring for Stephen with chronic disease alone
- possible financial difficulty
- consideration of going back to work
- more frequent consultations for minor illness in the future

Mr. Lee

- increased financial burden
- question of custody for Stephen
- possibility of casual sexual relations and risk of venereal disease
- living alone, lack of family support

Risk of alcohol or drug abuse for both Mr. and Mrs. Lee

Stephen

- risk of child abuse or overprotection
- asthma may become more difficult to control
- increased risk of behavioural problems
- lack of father at home may affect psychological or intellectual development

Doctor

- increased work load
- doctor dependence from patients

Index